The OCD Workbook

Your Step-by-Step Treatment Manual to Understand, Manage and Overcome Obsessive-Compulsive Disorder

Mila von Leiem

Table of Contents

Introduction

Congratulations on purchasing *The OCD Workbook,* and thank you for doing so.

The following chapters will discuss Obsessive-Compulsive Disorder in the context of a self-help workbook. We'll start by exploring what OCD is and what causes it. Afterward, we'll detail the different therapies and strategies used in the treatment of OCD, such as Exposure and Response Prevention Therapy, Cognitive Therapy, Acceptance and Commitment Therapy, cognitive diffusion, and mindfulness. In each chapter, we will provide a brief overview of the therapy. However, our primary focus will be to show you how to implement these techniques into your everyday life.

We will also discuss different subtypes of OCD, such as hyper-responsibility, compulsive hoarding, hypochondriasis, and the treatments specific to those conditions. Mental health conditions often associated with OCD, such as depression and anxiety, will also be discussed.

At the end of the book is a chapter containing additional resources to help you on your journey. If you need help finding a good therapist or locating support groups, this is the place to start.

To finish things off, we have included an additional chapter to help family members support loved ones who have been diagnosed with OCD.

Living with OCD can be a long and winding road, but you don't have to walk it alone. We hope that you will be able to utilize the information and techniques in this book to break the cycle of your obsessions and compulsions and live your best life.

There are plenty of books on this subject on the market, and we are so glad you let us take this journey with you!

Chapter 1: How to Get the Most Out of This Book

Before we get into the nitty-gritty details, we wanted to talk a little more about this book's structure. We'll keep it short and sweet since we already outlined *OCD Workbook* in the Introduction.

The book itself is divided into four sections:

The first part will introduce the topic of Obsessive-Compulsive Disorder. In this section, we will discuss what OCD is, its symptoms, causes, and how it is diagnosed.

The chapters that follow in section two are the core of our self-help guide. Chapters 5 through 10 feature different therapies and strategies used to treat OCD. Each section will start with a brief overview of the treatment. However, most of the chapter will focus on putting the techniques and skills covered into practice.

To this end, specific chapters may include quick reference guides or interactive worksheets for your review. The worksheets are designed to help you build your personalized plan and monitor your progress as you work through the book. We encourage you to experiment with each of the techniques to find the ones that work best for you.

Section three (chapters 11 through 14) will discuss different subtypes of OCD and mental health conditions commonly associated with OCD. Chapters 11 through 13 will feature hyper-responsibility, compulsive hoarding, and hypochondriasis, respectively. Each section will start with a brief introduction of the topic, followed by the therapies and techniques commonly used to treat each condition. Recommendations for additional readings/resources are included where appropriate.

Chapter 14 will feature mental health conditions associated with OCD. As anxiety is a critical component of OCD, chapter 13 will predominantly focus on anxiety disorders and their management.

The last section will comprise chapters 16 and 17. In chapter 16, Getting Help, you will find recommendations for additional resources to help you on your journey. The International OCD Organization, for example, provides access to online resource directories that you can use to find a therapist, clinic, or support group near your location. If you need a therapist or support group, this is an excellent place to start.

Chapter 17 includes resources for the family members and loved ones of those diagnosed with OCD. Individuals with the condition may also find this chapter a helpful reference when deciding how to talk about the subject with their loved ones.

Please note that this book is designed to be a self-help guide. It should not replace the psychiatric or psychological treatment of a licensed mental health professional. If you are in crisis or feel like you need help, please reach out to your medical provider or see our chapter on Getting Help for additional resources.

The best way to use this book is in conjunction with the treatment of a licensed mental health professional. It may also be used by those reluctant to seek professional help or those without access to a mental health professional such as a Psychiatrist, Psychologist, therapist, etc. If possible, we highly recommend seeking out the advice and treatment of a qualified professional.

OCD is a chronic mental health condition with no definitive cure. With the proper treatment, however, people with OCD can lead happy and fulfilling lives. We hope that by using the treatments and strategies in this book, you will have the tools necessary to break the cycle of your obsessions and compulsions and to lead your best life.

Chapter 2: What is OCD?

What is Obsessive-Compulsive Disorder

According to the Diagnostic and Statistical Manual of Mental Disorders (American Psychiatric Association 2000), Obsessive-Compulsive Disorder is considered part of a class of psychiatric disorders known as anxiety disorders. Other anxiety disorders include generalized anxiety disorder, social anxiety, post-traumatic stress disorder, and panic disorder.

Once believed to be rare, OCD is more common than initially thought, affecting approximately 1 out of every 40 people. Additionally, many with OCD are ashamed or embarrassed by their condition and try to "hide it" as a result. In recent years, however, there has been an increase in public awareness and acceptance of mental health conditions. This, along with advances in our understanding of OCD, has prompted many to come forward. Despite increased awareness, however, stigmatization and ignorance of OCD and psychiatric disorders, in general, persists in certain areas of society. As a result, some with OCD may still be reluctant to seek professional help and often don't get the treatment they need for their disorder.

Defining OCD

Obsessive-Compulsive Disorder is characterized by obsessions and compulsions that are distressing, time-consuming, and interfere with a person's ability to function. The obsessions and compulsions may interfere with the individual's relationships and social functioning.

OCD affects everyone equally, regardless of gender, race, or ethnicity. While OCD can occur at any age from preschool into adulthood, it usually first appears during the period from late childhood into adolescence or during the period from the late teens to early twenties. Additionally, males are more likely to develop OCD in childhood or adolescence, and females are more likely to experience onset in their twenties.

Interestingly, research shows that the age of onset may influence an individual's response to treatment and the symptoms they experience. For example, individuals with early-onset OCD (before the age of ten) may experience more severe symptoms than those with late-onset OCD (onset at age ten or older.) Symptoms also tend to develop gradually in early-onset OCD and more suddenly in late-onset OCD. The sudden manifestation of symptoms in late-onset OCD may be associated with a triggering event, such as a loved one's death or loss of a job. It is also not uncommon for women to experience the onset of OCD during pregnancy.

Those with early-onset OCD may also find it more difficult to find a treatment plan which works for them. For some, this may entail trying multiple treatment regimens, which may or may not include medications, Cognitive Behavioral Therapy, etc.

It's important to note that while a stressful event may act as a trigger for OCD, it does not cause OCD. The stressor merely facilitates the development of the disorder in a susceptible individual. Similarly, pregnancy does not cause OCD, but it can trigger the condition in a predisposed woman. Women previously diagnosed with OCD may experience a worsening of their symptoms during a pregnancy; however, many women report no changes in their symptoms while pregnant.

Obsessions and Compulsions

Obsessive thoughts and compulsive behaviors are more common than you might think. Most people will experience one or the other at some point in their lives. However, this doesn't mean that everyone with obsessions and compulsions has Obsessive-Compulsive Disorder. For the diagnosis of OCD to be considered, the cycle of obsessions and compulsions must be severe enough to impair a person's ability to function and perform their everyday activities. The distressing and time-consuming nature of the obsessions and compulsions may interfere with the individual's social life and place strain on relationships.

Obsessive Thoughts and Urges

The words "obsessive" and "obsessed" are used quite often in our day-to-day conversations. Think of the teenage girl, for example, who is "obsessed" with the latest boy band. In this context, the word obsessive has an almost pleasurable quality to it. The young girl's fixation with the boy band doesn't cause her distress. On the contrary, thinking about the band makes her quite happy. These thoughts don't interfere with her ability to go to school, socialize with friends, etc.

Compare this to the individual with Obsessive-Compulsive Disorder. For those with OCD, obsessions are characterized by repetitive, intrusive thoughts, images, or impulses. Often, the thoughts cause profound distress and feelings of disgust, anxiety, fear, or doubt. In many cases, individuals with OCD recognize that these thoughts don't make any sense; however, they feel powerless to control them.

Given the feelings of distress and anxiety associated with their obsessions, individuals often try to suppress their thoughts or neutralize them with another thought or action (compulsion). By engaging in ritualized thoughts and behaviors, the person finds temporary relief from their obsessions. Unfortunately, these compulsive behaviors are not a solution to the problem and can be just as problematic as the obsessions themselves.

The most common obsessions encountered in OCD generally fall into one of the following categories: contamination, losing control, harm, obsessions related to perfectionism, unwanted sexual thoughts, religious obsessions, hoarding, health obsessions, and miscellaneous obsessions.

Contamination: Contamination revolves around the fear of becoming seriously ill following perceived exposure to a contaminant, disease, or hazardous material. We say "perceived exposure" as, even though the individual was not physically exposed, they are convinced in their mind that they were exposed.

Additionally, the individual may live with the fear of causing harm to another if they fail to prevent the exposure from occurring. To relieve their anxiety they may engage in excessive washing and cleaning. Over time, the washing and cleaning rituals may become more complex and often provide less relief.

Take the case of a man, for example, who believed that his hands had become contaminated after touching a doorknob. Even though his hands were free from any visible contaminants, he was convinced that his hands were dirty, resulting in excessive handwashing. Over time, he began associating other objects with germs and contamination and began spending more time washing his hands each day. The handwashing became so frequent that he developed a red, itchy, scaly rash over both of his hands.

Other sources of perceived contamination include germs, dirt, household chemicals, environmental contaminants (radon, asbestos, radiation, toxic waste), animals, insects, diseases (STDs, HIV, herpes, hepatitis,) and bodily fluids.

Fear of Losing Control: Fear of losing control is another prominent obsession in OCD and can take on many forms. One individual may have a fear of acting on an impulse to harm themselves or to harm others. In contrast, another individual may have a fear of blurting out obscenities or insults. Note that while the individual may be having these thoughts, they would rather *not* have them given the distress associated with them.

Harm: Another frequently encountered obsession is the fear of causing harm to other people. Often, the fear stems from the belief that if the individual isn't careful enough in performing a task or fails to complete a task, they will be directly responsible for harming another person. For example, consider the case of an individual who experiences frequent urges to check that his stove is off. These urges are driven by the belief that if he fails to do so, it will start a house fire, resulting in the injury or death of his family.

Perfectionism: Obsessions related to perfectionism are some of the most widely recognized manifestations of OCD. Individuals who experience perfection-related obsessions may be overly concerned with symmetry and orderliness. For example, think of the person who organized the books in their bookcase until they are "just right."

Sexual Obsessions: Unwanted sexual thoughts are some of the most distressing obsessions experienced by people with OCD. The sexual thoughts or images may involve forbidden or taboo subjects such as aggressive sexual behavior, incest, or pedophilia. These thoughts do not reflect the sexual preferences or tendencies of the person. On the contrary, these individuals often experience feelings of extreme perturbation or disgust with these obsessions. The distress may become so severe that the person may try to avoid contact with the person or persons that trigger the obsession. Not surprisingly, this can put a strain on relationships and lead to social isolation.

Religious Obsessions: Religious obsessions vary depending on one's culture and religious beliefs. Those who experience religious obsessions may exhibit an excessive concern with morality and fear of committing blasphemy. Fear of blaspheming is more common among those with strong religious beliefs, such as Catholics and Orthodox Jews.

To combat these fears, individuals may engage in elaborate prayers or seek reassurance from other people.

Hoarding: Those with hoarding obsessions exhibit an urge to collect seemingly useless things that others might consider "junk." The thought of getting rid of the item often causes significant distress. As a result, they keep the object, believing that they may need it in the future. Additionally, those with hoarding obsessions may have the urge to buy multiples of the same item.

This accumulation of items can result in chaotic (and potentially unsafe) living conditions as the objects gradually take up more and more space in the home, apartment, etc.

Health Obsessions: Health-related obsessions involve excessive preoccupation or fear of having a severe illness. This belief is maintained even after the person is reassured that they are completely healthy. They may also believe themselves responsible for causing the affliction of a loved one.

Miscellaneous Obsessions: Lastly, obsessions may involve superstitious ideas such as specific numbers, words, or colors being lucky or unlucky. They may also have an excessive fear of making mistakes, losing things, or have an undesired urge to remember useless information such as license plates, names, words, etc.

Compulsive Behaviors

Compulsions are repetitive thoughts or behaviors that people use to neutralize or counteract their obsessions. Any relief gained from performing the compulsive thought or action is temporary as the obsessions inevitably reoccur over time. Often, people with OCD don't have a better means of coping with their obsessions and continue to rely on their compulsions as a means of temporary escape. Over time, an individual's compulsions may become more complex while paradoxically providing less relief.

As with obsessions, the context in which repetitive or ritualized behaviors occur matters. Religious services, for example, may also involve repetitive behaviors or rituals. Similarly, your morning routine may consist of a set schedule that you repeat every day without fail. While both involve repetitive actions, they don't necessarily fall under the category of OCD-related behaviors. Your morning routine is a set part of your schedule and likely wouldn't interfere with your other daily activities.

In contrast, compulsions are often time-consuming and interfere with essential activities in a person's everyday life. Additionally, while compulsions provide temporary relief from obsessions, individuals with OCD typically don't derive pleasure from performing them. Most people would prefer not to engage in these repetitive thoughts and behaviors. However, they feel compelled to do so because of the distress associated with their obsessions.

Common compulsions in OCD include washing/cleaning, checking, repeating/counting/ordering, hoarding, health-related and mental compulsions.

Washing: Washing may involve excessive hand washing, showering/bathing, grooming, or tooth brushing. In particular, excessive hand washing can lead to the development of dry, cracked, scaly rashes on the surface of the hands, known as contact dermatitis. Individuals may also engage in excessive cleaning of household items or other objects to prevent contact with perceived contaminants.

Checking: Checking related compulsions may involve checking to ensure that the doors and windows are locked, the stove is off, etc. For example, consider an individual who feels compelled to repeatedly check their kitchen and bathroom sinks to ensure they aren't running. This compulsion is driven by the fear that failure to do so will result in their house flooding with water. To prevent this event from happening, they repeatedly get up throughout the night to check both of their sinks. While performing this compulsion provides them with temporary relief, it is also highly disruptive and negatively impacts their ability to get a good night's sleep.

Additionally, checking related compulsions may prompt someone with OCD to repeatedly check that they didn't cause harm to themselves or someone else. For example, one individual with OCD became convinced that he had hit someone with his car by accident. Consequently, he began to frantically drive the same route over and over again to make sure that he hadn't seriously injured or killed someone.

Repeating/Counting/Ordering: Compulsions may also involve repeating specific movements or activities.

Individuals may feel compelled to repeatedly blink or touch an object a certain number of times. Additionally, they may repeat routine activities or tasks a certain number of times. An example of a repetitive compulsion would be going in or out of a door four times because four is a "good" number.

Individuals may also count objects or count during other compulsive activities such as washing/cleaning or checking.

Ordering generally involves arranging objects in a particular order or until it feels "just right." For example, an individual with an ordering obsession might arrange the pens on their desk in a neat line from largest to smallest.

Hoarding: Hoarding involves the collection of seemingly useless items that other people might consider "junk." The thought of throwing the object away often causes significant distress, prompting the individual to keep the item believing that it may prove useful in the future.

Health-Related Compulsions: Health-related compulsions can be especially time-consuming. The fear of having a severe illness may prompt individuals with health-related obsessions to seek reassurance and may result in unnecessary medical tests. Individuals may also spend excessive amounts of time checking their body for signs of disease (such as taking their blood pressure or heart rate) or researching the disease online.

Mental Compulsions: Mental compulsions may involve counting while performing an activity to end on a "good" number. Similarly, individuals may use a "good" word or thought to cancel out a "bad" word or thought. To prevent harm or prevent something terrible from happening, people may also perform mental reviews of events.

Other miscellaneous compulsions include actively avoiding situations that might trigger an obsession, excessively seeking reassurance from others, and an excessive need to confess wrong behavior.

How Is OCD Diagnosed?

Only a qualified medical or mental health professional such as a psychiatrist or psychologist can make the diagnosis of Obsessive-Compulsive Disorder. To meet the diagnostic criteria, the individual must have obsessions and compulsions that are time-consuming and interfere with their ability to perform essential activities such as working, going to school, and socializing with friends and family.

During the initial assessment, the severity of the individual's OCD is also assessed. This step is essential as the level of severity reflects the degree to which the person's OCD interferes with their lives and helps guide the treatment plan. Assessment of the severity of the individual's condition usually involves an OCD scale.

The most commonly used scale is the Yale-Brown Obsessive-Compulsive Scale I and II (Y-BOCS I and Y-BOCS II). To assess OCD severity in children there is a Children's Yale-Brown Obsessive-Compulsive Scale (CY-BOCS). The scale consists of 10 questions, with each item ranging from 0 to 4 points depending on severity. The final score ranges from 0 to 40 points, with 0 being the least severe and 40 the most severe.

The questionnaire assesses OCD severity based on five categories:

1. Amount of time spent on obsessions and compulsions.

2. The degree to which the obsessions and compulsions interfere with everyday life.

3. Level of distress caused by the obsessions and compulsions.

4. The individual's ability to resist their obsessions and compulsions.

5. How much control the individual has over their obsessions and compulsions.

The Chronic Nature of OCD

Obsessive-Compulsive Disorder is a lifelong condition and tends to vary in severity throughout one's life. Symptoms may be mild to moderate or so severe that they impair a person's ability to function. It's not uncommon for symptoms to become more severe during times of great stress. Additionally, the types of obsessions and compulsions experienced may vary throughout life as well.

Naturally, many of the treatments for OCD will vary depending on the severity of your symptoms, obsessions, and compulsions. Therefore, to get the most out of the following chapters, it may help to assess the severity of your OCD first.

The Yale-Brown Obsessive-Compulsive Scale is the most widely recognized OCD scale and is easily found online. It's only ten questions and can be completed relatively quickly. To monitor your progress it may be helpful to fill out the questionnaire before starting the program, approximately half-way through the program, and at the end of the program. This will allow you to gauge your progress as you work through the self-help guide.

Before creating a treatment plan, it may also be helpful to identify your obsessions and compulsions. To this end, we have included a worksheet in the pages that follow.

Take a moment to fill out the worksheet "Identifying Your Obsessions and Compulsions" before moving on to the next chapter.

Identifying Your Obsessions and Compulsions

Take a moment to think about your obsessions and compulsions. Was there something that triggered the obsession? What emotions did you experience when the obsessive thought or urge occurred? What coping mechanism or compulsion did you use?

Below you will find a table where you can jot down your responses. After filling out the worksheet, take a moment to consider how your OCD has impacted your life. How has it impacted your ability to function at work/school? How has it affected your relationships?

Trigger What occurred before you experienced the obsessive thought/urge?	Obsession Intrusive thought, image, or urge	Emotions Experienced What did you feel?	Compulsion/ Coping Strategy What did you do?

Chapter 3: What Causes OCD?

Despite recent advances in both science and medicine over the past several decades, there is still a lot that we don't know about Obsessive-Compulsive Disorder. Numerous factors are believed to contribute to the development of OCD, including neurobiological, genetic, cognitive, behavioral, and environmental factors. The degree to which each of these contributes to the development of the disorder is unknown.

Neurobiological Theories

Using neuroimaging studies to take "pictures" of the brain, researchers have determined that some brain regions function differently in those with OCD compared to those without the disorder. In particular, communication between the orbitofrontal complex, the caudate nucleus of the basal ganglia, and the thalamus are impaired.

The orbitofrontal complex is responsible for reward-based decision-making and goal-directed behavior. It also helps regulate our ability to control our emotions. The caudate nucleus plays a vital role in our ability to think, learn, and perform voluntary muscle movements.

Communication between these structures is analogous to a circuit in which the different brain areas "talk" to each other through neural impulses. When these circuits are activated, a thought or urge is brought to your attention. When this occurs, your brain then prompts you to act to address this impulse. In OCD, it's theorized that this circuit becomes hyperactive, resulting in the obsessions and compulsions characteristic of the disorder.

This theory is supported by neuroimaging findings which have shown abnormal activity within brain structures involved in this circuit, such as the orbitofrontal complex and caudate nucleus. Essentially, this suggests that people with OCD may have difficulty "turning off" these impulses or may be unable to turn them off altogether. Research has also shown that treatments for OCD such as Cognitive Behavioral Therapy and medications help normalize activity within this circuit.

The Serotonin System

Serotonin is a chemical messenger (neurotransmitter) used by our brain to transmit a message from one nerve cell to another. It helps regulate our mood and sleep cycle. Low levels of serotonin have been linked with depression, anxiety, and insomnia.

Not surprisingly, antidepressants such as selective serotonin reuptake inhibitors (SSRIs) are used to treat depression and anxiety disorders. SSRIs act by preventing the reabsorption of serotonin in the brain so that more of it remains active.

Interestingly, SSRIs have proven effective in the treatment of OCD as well. While we don't know precisely why SSRIs are effective for OCD, it's hypothesized that low levels of serotonin within the brain may contribute to the development of OCD.

It should be noted that while most individuals experience a reduction in their symptoms, others derive minimal relief from these medications. In some cases, additional drugs may be needed to enhance the effectiveness of the first-line medication. Therefore, while low levels of serotonin may contribute to OCD, it is not the only cause.

Genetics

Studies suggest that there may be a genetic component to OCD as well; however, the exact genes involved are not known. Statistically, you are more likely to develop OCD if you have a family member with the condition. In fact, around 25% of people with OCD have at least one close family member with the disorder. OCD which develops in childhood also appears to have a more substantial genetic component than OCD which develops later in life.

Cognitive-Behavioral Theories

Cognitive-Behavioral Theory views OCD through the lens of a learned process. People who are predisposed to OCD experience unwanted, intrusive thoughts often over the course of the day. While most people would be able to brush such thoughts aside, individuals with OCD cannot do so.

For example, let's say you keep experiencing the sudden thought that you might hit your friend. This thought leaves you feeling understandably distressed. Part of you may even fear that you may act on this impulse and harm your friend. As a result, this thought becomes dangerous in your mind. Every time the thought surfaces, you become hyper-aware of it. Before long, it becomes difficult to focus on anything else, and the thought becomes an obsession.

Compulsions may also be a learned process. A classic example that Cognitive-Behavioral Theorists use is that of handwashing. Upon experiencing the feeling of contamination (the obsession in this case), you might wash your hands. After performing this action (the compulsion), your anxiety may temporarily improve. Even though you know the obsession will come back, the temporary relief from your anxiety is enough to reinforce this behavior. Every time you experience this particular obsession, therefore, you respond with the same compulsion.

Through this vicious cycle, Obsessive-Compulsive Disorder is born. Keep in mind that this is a theory, and there is still much about OCD that we don't know.

Environment

Environmental factors and stressors such as childhood trauma have been linked with the development of OCD. As discussed previously, the stressors or traumatic events themselves don't cause OCD. Still, they may act as a trigger in a susceptible individual.

PANDAS/PANS

Pediatric Autoimmune Neuropsychiatric Disorder Associated with Streptococcus (PANDAS) is the sudden onset of obsessive-compulsive behavior in a child following infection with *Streptococcus pyogenes*, commonly referred to as "Strep." The age of onset varies;

however, most children who develop PANDAS (or PANS) are between 3 and 14 years old.

The condition develops rapidly and is sometimes referred to as "overnight OCD" for that reason. In addition to the obsessions and compulsions that develop, children may also experience "tics" or other repetitive, purposeless movements. Sudden changes in mood and ADHD-type symptoms such as difficulty concentrating, hyperactivity, and the inability to sit still have also been reported. Additionally, children may exhibit extreme separation anxiety, changes in fine motor skills (especially handwriting), and changes in sleep patterns as well.

Strep isn't the only infection that can provoke the onset of OCD symptoms in a child. Recent research has shown that infection with Mycoplasma pneumonia, Epstein Barr (mono), Lyme disease, Varicella (chickenpox), Herpes simplex, and the flu virus can cause these symptoms as well. In this case, the condition is known as Pediatric Acute-onset Neuropsychiatric Syndrome (PANS).

While the exact reason for this is unknown, it's believed that the child's immune system may mistakenly attack certain areas of the brain rather than the infection. The result is the sudden onset of OCD symptoms in a child that was healthy and happy only days before. In contrast, the onset of OCD in childhood (that is not provoked by an infection) is usually gradual.

Not every child who develops one of the infections listed above will go on to develop PANDAS or PANS. If you suspect your child may have PANDAS or PANS, you should immediately get in touch with your child's Pediatrician. Your Pediatrician will evaluate your child for infection and provide treatment as appropriate. Treatment of the OCD/behavioral component of PANDAS/PANS often requires a specialist. If you are interested in learning more about these conditions, you can find additional resources in chapters 16 and 17.

Chapter 4: Overview of Treatment Options

Treatment for OCD includes medications, psychotherapy, or a combination of the two. In most cases, a combination of the two therapies is used and often produces the best results. Medications should only be used to treat OCD under the direction of a qualified mental health professional. Therefore, as medications are beyond the scope of this self-help guide, we will be focusing on the different therapies and techniques used to treat OCD. If you have questions about the role of medications in the treatment of OCD, please refer to chapter 16, Getting Help, or get in touch with a local mental health professional.

With all of the treatments available for OCD, it's easy to get lost trying to find the option that works best for you. Fortunately, we'll be going over the most commonly used therapies and techniques used to treat OCD. We'll start by covering Exposure and Response Prevention Therapy (ERP), the most widely used and perhaps most successful treatment for OCD. Afterward, we'll take a look at traditional Cognitive Therapy (CT), followed by Acceptance and Commitment Therapy (ACT). To finish things off, we'll take a quick look at two powerful techniques known as cognitive diffusion and mindfulness that can be used to support you on your journey.

Treatment options for different aspects of OCD, such as hyper-responsibility, compulsive hoarding, and hypochondriasis, will be covered in their respective chapters. Given the nature of compulsive hoarding and hypochondriasis, treatment strategies for these conditions may differ from those used to treat Obsessive-Compulsive Disorder in general. Therefore, the specific treatments used for compulsive hoarding and hypochondriasis are covered separately.

Conditions associated with OCD, such as anxiety, will also be covered in later chapters. In particular, we'll consider the role of Dialectical Behavioral Therapy (DBT) in the treatment of anxiety.

Quick reference sheets and worksheets will be provided in specific chapters where appropriate. The worksheets are designed to help you create your personalized treatment plan and to monitor your progress as you work through the self-help program.

Individual responses to the treatments will vary depending on the severity of OCD symptoms and other factors such as adherence to the treatment plan and the presence of other mental health conditions. Therefore, we encourage you to experiment with the following treatment options to find the plan that works best for your individual needs. Coexisting mental health conditions such as depression and anxiety may need to be addressed individually and in some cases, by a qualified mental health professional.

As previously mentioned, this book is not meant to act as a substitute for the treatment of a qualified medical professional. We highly recommend using this book in conjunction with the treatment of a licensed mental health professional to get the best results. Some of the treatments in this self-help guide may cause feelings of discomfort, anxiety, and distress. This is part of the treatment process and a necessary step towards your recovery. Having the support of a mental health professional during these critical periods can be extremely beneficial and help keep you on track. If you are reluctant to seek treatment from a licensed professional or do not have access to one, recruiting a friend or loved one to act as a source of support may help.

If you choose to recruit a friend or a loved one, we encourage them to read the book as well. This will give them a better understanding of what OCD is and how it is treated. By understanding the treatment process, they will also be able to provide you with the support you need.

Chapter 5: Exposure and Response Prevention Therapy

Exposure and Response Prevention Therapy (ERP) is a type of Cognitive Behavioral Therapy (CBT) that involves exposing an individual to a situation to provoke an obsession. The goal of ERP is to help the person cope with the distress and anxiety associated with an obsession while preventing them from engaging in their normal, compulsive responses. In essence, ERP forces you to face your fears and teaches you to handle the discomfort associated with them without engaging in unhelpful coping strategies (compulsions).

For example, a woman with a fear of contamination might be asked to pick up a used tissue and hold it in her hand for an hour. During this time, she wouldn't be allowed to engage in her normal compulsive behaviors such as handwashing.

Similarly, a person who experiences sudden, distressing thoughts of inflicting harm on other people might be asked to spend extended periods with family and friends and would be prohibited from self-isolating. In each case, the form of ERP varies depending on the individual's obsessions and compulsions.

Think this sounds a bit extreme? Well, you wouldn't be alone in that thought. The concept of therapy, something that should be healing in nature, intentionally putting someone through such pain seems wrong. Moreover, why would people intentionally subject themselves to this? Surely, there has to be a better way?

While it's true that there are other treatments for OCD, ERP is among the most widely used and the most effective. Indeed, research has shown ERP to be highly effective not just for OCD but for Social Anxiety Disorder, Panic Disorder, Phobias, and Post Traumatic Stress Disorder as well. But why is this?

As it turns out, the short term discomfort associated with ERP is well worth the long term gain. And as advocates of ERP will tell you, the pain associated with the therapy is usually minuscule compared to the prolonged suffering of those with untreated OCD.

With that being said, ERP isn't easy. Rather than avoid your obsessions, you will be asked to confront them and the discomfort associated with them. The key to success in ERP is to allow yourself to experience the triggered thoughts, images, and emotions, however unpleasant they might be, and refrain from engaging in your compulsive responses.

In this chapter, we will guide you through the process of ERP. Additionally, at the end of the chapter, you will find a worksheet to help you build your own ERP plan. Please note that some level of discomfort is to be expected with ERP. If, at any time, however, your distress becomes too great, don't be afraid to scale back the difficulty of your plan. Having a mental health professional, friend, or family member as a source of support can be very helpful.

Setting Realistic Goals

The first and perhaps most critical step of ERP is to set realistic goals for yourself. Start with the obsessions that are least distressing to you and work your way up from there. Success with Exposure and Response Prevention Therapy doesn't happen overnight. Starting small is more likely to lead to success further down the road.

Making a list of your obsessions from least to most distressing can be helpful. Again, if you feel that a particular obsession is causing too much distress, take a step back, and consider taking on a different obsession. You can always come back to that obsession later.

Lastly, don't get discouraged if you don't notice a change right away. All treatments take time. While many individuals notice a difference after the first couple of sessions, it may take longer for others to see a benefit.

Exposure Therapy

After selecting an obsession to challenge, you're ready to move on to the next step – facing your fears. Confronting fear can be a frightening prospect; however, many individuals with OCD report that it's not as distressing as they thought it would be once they start. Gradually, the obsessions lose their power over the individual and no longer trigger feelings of anxiety or distress. Ultimately, the obsessions become just like any other thought.

Ideally, ERP should be administered under the supervision of a qualified mental health professional when undertaken for the first time. However, finding a qualified professional to administer the therapy can be difficult and, in some cases, costly. Additionally, some individuals may be reluctant to seek professional help.

One of the benefits of ERP is that individuals can practice self-directed exposure and response prevention exercises at times and locations convenient to them.

The number of sessions required will vary depending on the individual and the challenge imposed by the obsession. Obsessions that cause more distress will take more time to conquer. Expect to set aside 60 to 90 minutes per session to start. When conducted under the supervision of a therapist, individuals typically undergo 2 to 5 sessions per week. Therefore, make sure you are practicing your ERP exercises several times per week.

Remember that adherence to your ERP plan is critical. One of the most common reasons for treatment failure is due to individuals dropping out before reaching the end of their program.

Imaginal Exposure

When beginning ERP for the first time, it may help to start by imaging the exposure in your mind. Mentally confronting the trigger can help desensitize you to its effects before attempting to face it in real life. Imaginal exposure can be particularly helpful if you anticipate the trigger will cause significant distress.

Imaginal exposure isn't limited to visualizing the trigger in your head. Writing out the content of your obsession or making an audio recording can be particularly helpful for certain people. In this case, exposure consists of reading or listening to your statement. This is repeated until you begin to experience some measure of relief from your symptoms.

For example, a woman who is plagued by thoughts of injuring her father might be asked to make a detailed audio recording in which she describes these thoughts in detail. The exposure would consist of her listening to this recording until she experiences a reduction in the anxiety provoked by this thought.

Graduated Exposure

Gradually increasing your exposure to a trigger may also be beneficial. This is known as the "slow as you go approach," where the intensity of exposure is increased over time. For example, an individual with a fear of contamination might be asked to touch an object with their index finger. Over subsequent exposures, they would be asked to touch the object with two fingers, three fingers, etc. The level of contact with the object would be increased until their entire hand was in contact with the object.

Shaping

Keep in mind that this process takes time. When visualizing a trigger or confronting it in real life, you may not experience a decrease in your symptoms right away. Some individuals may find that it takes an hour or more before their distress begins to abate. When planning an ERP session, therefore, make sure that you have enough time set aside. Sessions may take 60 minutes or more but shouldn't be longer than 90 minutes.

Once the session begins, it's essential to follow it through to the end. Stopping before you experience relief from your symptoms will render the treatment ineffective. Additionally, stopping early or giving in to your compulsive responses may reinforce the power your obsessions and compulsions have over you. Ideally, the session should continue until you experience at least a 50% reduction in your anxiety.

As difficult as it may be, you must push through the discomfort for the treatment to be effective. When you first notice the distress, don't suppress it. Acknowledge it's presence. Take note of what you are feeling at that moment in time.

What thoughts are going through your mind? Are you experiencing any physical symptoms? If so, take note of them as well.

Most people will notice a gradual increase in their distress, which levels off after a few minutes. The distressing sensations then diminish slowly, over time. Once your feelings of discomfort start to decrease, your mind is beginning to reap the benefits of the therapy. Gradually, over time, your mind learns that there is nothing to fear from the trigger. With each session, you will find that your distress level decreases until you have little or no reaction to the trigger. This process is known as shaping and is a critical component of the treatment process.

Breaking the Cycle of Obsessions and Compulsions

For ERP to be genuinely effective, confronting the content of your obsessions is not enough. You must also refrain from engaging in your compulsive thoughts and behaviors.

For some, this can be the most challenging aspect of ERP. While compulsions do provide some measure of relief from your obsessions, that relief is temporary. Inevitably the obsession will come back. Performing a compulsive ritual won't change that. It also won't help you learn to deal with your obsessions in the long run.

Not all compulsions may be as obvious as handwashing or checking your windows four times to make sure they're locked. Sometimes people don't even realize they are engaging in compulsive behaviors.

Distraction and avoidance are very common ways people try to "cope" with their obsessions. Distraction, in particular, is one of the first things many people use to deal with their obsessions. Rather than face the discomfort and anxiety associated with their obsession, they will try to keep themselves busy, put on some music, watch tv, etc. By focusing their mind on something else, they actively avoid dealing with their obsessions. And as we know, avoiding a problem isn't an effective way to deal with it.

Avoidance provides a similar means of relief from obsessions. Like distraction, however, the relief is temporary. By distracting yourself or avoiding the obsession altogether, you prevent yourself from confronting the obsession and the discomfort associated with it. Thus, the vicious cycle is allowed to continue. Only by facing your obsessive thoughts and urges can you break the cycle and find relief from your symptoms.

Reassurance is another way people with OCD seek relief from their anxiety. Paradoxically, however, the more reassurance a person with OCD receives, the more comfort they seek out. Reassurance, after all, only provides short term relief and does not address the underlying issue. Additionally, a person's constant requests for reassurance can strain their relationships with friends and loved ones.

While it can be challenging, the key is to not seek reassurance as a means of coping with your obsessions. To this end, it may be helpful to educate your friends and family members about the harmful effects of reassurance on the recovery process. If you're not sure where to start, have them read this chapter. Chapter 17, Resources for Family Members, may also be helpful.

In the event you do try to seek reassurance, make sure they know not to provide any. This may seem harsh, but it is crucial for your recovery in the long run. Creating a gentle refusal statement for them may be beneficial. For example, they might say something to the effect of: "It sounds like you are asking for reassurance. Remember that reassurance is not helpful and can be harmful."

How to Handle Set-Backs

Many people will experience set-backs and relapses during the treatment process. No one is perfect, after all, as much as we would like to think otherwise. Rather than view these experiences as a failure, it's important to think of them as learning opportunities.

Let's say, for example, that you give in to your compulsion during a session. Rather than writing the entire session off as a failure, ask yourself, "Why did I give in to my compulsion? What prompted me to engage in this behavior? What can I do differently to prevent this from happening again?" Most importantly, however, reexpose yourself to the trigger and start over.

Creating Your Own ERP Plan

Now that we've covered the basics of ERP, it's time for you to create your own ERP plan. You will find an outline that you can use to build your personalized plan on the next few pages. A sample ERP plan has been provided for reference, as well. After the sample plan, you will find a chart that you can use to track your progress.

Remember, ERP is a gradual process. However, if you commit yourself to face your fears head-on, you *can* break the cycle of your obsessions and compulsions.

Creating an ERP Plan

The following worksheet can be used as a guide to create a personalized ERP plan. At the end of the worksheet, you will find a chart to document your progress over time. Remember that this is a gradual process, so don't get discouraged if you don't notice an improvement in your symptoms right away!

Step 1: Setting Realistic Goals

Make a list of your obsessions. Start with the obsession that is the least distressing and work your way up to the most uncomfortable. Ranking each obsession using a 0 –

10 numeric scale may be helpful. Take note of your list, as this is the order you will be completing them in.

Step 2: Imaginal Exposure/Exposure Therapy

Visualize the trigger in your mind to start. Writing down the content of your obsession or making an audio recording of yourself may also be helpful. When you feel you are ready, move on to confronting the trigger in real life. Pay close attention to what you are feeling, both emotionally and physically.

What feelings are you experiencing?
Are you experiencing any physical symptoms?

Step 3: Response Prevention

Refrain from giving in to your compulsive thoughts and behaviors. Don't try to distract yourself or avoid facing the trigger. Acknowledge both the trigger and the feelings and sensations that come with it. Remember, the short-term discomfort is well worth the long term gain of being freed from the cycle of your obsessions and compulsions! Don't seek reassurance either, as reassurance interferes with the recovery process. Continue the session until you experience at least a 50% reduction in your symptoms.

Step 4: Keep With It!

Try to be consistent with your sessions. Remember that sessions may take 60 minutes or longer, especially when first starting. Over time, you should notice a gradual decrease in your symptoms. By the end of treatment, the same triggers that were so distressing before should evoke little to no response.

Step 5: You Did It!

Congratulations, you made it! All that hard work has finally paid off, and you are one step closer to freeing yourself from the cycle of your obsessions and compulsions. With one obsession out of the way, it's time to move on to the next one.

Sample ERP Plan

Name Samuel M.

Step 1: Setting Realistic Goals

Make a list of your obsessions. Start with the obsession that is the least distressing and work your way up to the most uncomfortable. Ranking each obsession using a 0 – 10 numeric scale may be helpful. Take note of your list, as this is the order you will be completing them in.

Fear of becoming contaminated – from shaking hands with other people, coming into contact with surfaces frequently touched by other individuals such as doorknobs, etc.

My level of discomfort is 5/10.

Step 2: Imaginal Exposure/Exposure Therapy

Visualize the trigger in your mind to start. Writing the content of your obsession down or making an audio recording of yourself may also be helpful. When you feel you are ready, move on to confronting the trigger in real life. Pay close attention to what you are feeling, both emotionally and physically.

Imaginal Exposure*: I picture myself standing in the middle of a busy shopping center. Crowds of people filter in and out of the store around me. I approach the door to the shopping center. It isn't an automatic one, but one you have to pull to open.*

I begin to feel anxious, thinking of all the people who have touched this door handle. What if one of them was carrying some kind of illness? What if I get sick?

Rather than trying to think of something else, I acknowledge this thought and the anxiety that comes with it. In my mind, I see myself reach for the door handle and open it.

Almost immediately, I'm hit with the urge to wash my hands. My anxiety is building, but I force myself to wait. I let the uncomfortable feelings wash over me. As much as I don't want to experience them, I know I must do just that.

Gradually, the feeling of distress levels off then begins decreasing. I almost can't believe it, but sure enough, the anxiety continues to diminish.

What feelings are you experiencing?

At first, I felt extremely anxious, especially after I opened the door. I was afraid that I had become infected, and if I didn't wash my hands to cleanse myself, I would become very ill.

After 30 minutes or so, the feelings began to decrease until the anxiety became more manageable.

Are you experiencing any physical symptoms?

During my session, I felt like my heart was racing out of my chest. I even started sweating at one point. After a few minutes, however, these symptoms began to go away.

Exposure Therapy*: Once I feel confident that I can manage my distress when confronting my trigger mentally, I will move on to Exposure Therapy.*

During my exposure therapy session, I will visit a grocery store in person and open the door with my bare hands. Afterward, I will refrain from washing or sanitizing my hands in any way.

Step 3: Response Prevention

Refrain from giving in to your compulsive thoughts and behaviors. Don't try to distract yourself or avoid facing the trigger. Acknowledge both the trigger and the feelings and sensations that come with it. Remember, the short term discomfort is well worth the long term gain of being freed from the cycle of your obsessions and compulsions! Don't seek reassurance either, as reassurance interferes with the recovery process. Continue the session until you experience at least a 50% reduction in your symptoms.

After touching the door handle, I won't wash or sanitize my hands.

I won't seek reassurance from my sister either. My sister also knows not to reassure me.

Step 4: Keep With It!

Try to be consistent with your sessions. Remember that sessions may take 60 minutes or longer, especially when first starting. Over time, you should notice a gradual decrease in your symptoms. By the end of treatment, the same triggers that were so distressing before should evoke little to no response.

It's been several weeks, and I have noticed a steady decline in my symptoms. Initially, I was experiencing 5/10 discomfort. Now, however, my level of discomfort has decreased to 2/10.

Step 5: You Did It!

Congratulations, you made it! All that hard work has finally paid off, and you are one step closer to freeing yourself from the cycle of your obsessions and compulsions. With one obsession out of the way, it's time to move on to the next one.

When shaking hands or touching a surface that other people frequently come into contact with, I no longer have the urge to wash my hands. I rarely feel any anxiety at the thought of becoming contaminated. When I experience anxiety related to this, it is often so minuscule that I don't even notice.

Tracking Your Progress

Date	Exposure (Note if Imaginal or Real)	Discomfort (0 – 10) Beginning of Session	Feelings/Emotions	Physical Symptoms	Discomfort (0 – 10) End of Session

Chapter 6: Challenging Your Beliefs and the Role of Habituation

Challenging your beliefs is the first step on the road to breaking free from your obsessions and compulsions. By actively engaging in ERP, you will learn to cope with your obsessions and anxiety in a healthy manner, without resorting to your compulsions for temporary relief. The process by which this occurs is known as habituation.

Habituation

In the context of ERP, habituation refers to the reduction in anxiety and distress you experience with time. This means that through time and repeated exposure, your body learns that there is nothing to fear from your obsessions. As time progresses, your anxiety continues to diminish until it goes away entirely or becomes barely noticeable.

Given this information, you might ask, "Why doesn't habituation occur naturally?" Say you have an irrational fear of toaster ovens, for example. Every time you see a toaster oven, you are sent into a frenzied state of panic. If repeated exposure to something over time reduces the fear associated with it, you should, theoretically, become less and less terrified of toaster ovens every time you see one. In reality, however, your anxiety does not go away every time you see a toaster oven. But why is this?

The answer is that for habituation to truly work, you have to expose yourself to the dreaded trigger until your anxiety decreases or resolves altogether. This process takes time and, in some cases, may take an hour or more.

In most cases, when we are exposed to a trigger, our instinctive reaction is to run away or to avoid situations that expose us to the trigger altogether. The process of running away or avoiding the trigger, however, can create a negative reinforcement effect and can increase the amount of fear you experience when exposed to the trigger in the future.

In ERP, there are two types of habituation to consider. The first is called within-trial habituation, and the second is known as between-trial habituation.

Within-Trial Habituation

Within-trial, habituation refers to the reduction in anxiety you experience during a trial or treatment. For example, during an ERP session, within-trial habituation is the distress relief you experience during exposure to a trigger.

Remember, the key to ERP is to expose yourself to the trigger long enough for you to experience a reduction in your anxiety. Otherwise, you won't receive any benefit from the therapy. The amount of time required to achieve this will vary depending on the challenge presented by the obsession, the number of previous ERP sessions for that particular trigger, etc. Ideally, you should continue the session until you get a 50% reduction in your peak anxiety.

Between-Trial Habituation

Between-trial habituation refers to the reduction in the peak anxiety you experience when you repeat the exposure exercise over time. In this case, peak anxiety is the maximum amount of anxiety experienced during the entire exposure session.

To illustrate this, let's go back to our example with the toaster oven. Upon exposure to the trigger, in this case, a toaster oven, the peak anxiety is the point at which you feel the most anxious. After multiple sessions, you note that you don't feel nearly as anxious as you did during your first session. Even when your anxiety is at its worst, it doesn't come close to what it was before. This is between-trial habituation at work.

Through repeated exposure, your peak anxiety will diminish over time. To achieve this effect, however, you need to be consistent in your sessions. Exposing yourself to a trigger once a week, for example, isn't likely to get you anywhere. The time it takes for between-trial habituation to develop will vary depending on the individual and the challenge presented by the exposure. Many individuals will notice a change after the first couple of sessions; however, it may take longer for other people to see a difference.

Why Don't Compulsions Result in Habituation?

In a sense, compulsions can provide the equivalent of within-trial habituation, in that they temporarily reduce the anxiety associated with an obsession. Remember, however, that this is a temporary fix and does not resolve the underlying problem. By engaging in your compulsion, you may be relieving your anxiety, but you are preventing yourself from facing your fear. To overcome your obsessions and compulsions, you must expose yourself to your obsessions and your fears until you notice a reduction in your anxiety and distress. Without this critical step, between-trial habituation cannot be achieved. In a sense, between-trial habituation can be thought of as a measure of treatment success.

This is what makes ERP so successful. By reducing your peak anxiety over time through repeated exposure, ERP provides long-term relief of OCD symptoms and effectively breaks the cycle of obsessions and compulsions. In fact, studies have shown that individuals who discontinue treatment with CBT are less likely to relapse than individuals who stop therapy with medication.

Is ERP More Effective Than Medications?

According to experts, ERP may be more effective in the treatment of OCD than medications. ERP has the additional benefit of being faster acting than medications as well. For example, individuals may notice an improvement in their symptoms after the first couple of ERP sessions. In comparison, individuals receiving medications may not see any improvement until ten to twelve weeks after starting the medicine.

However, this does not mean that there is no role for medications in the treatment of OCD. CBT, when used in conjunction with medication, is more effective than either therapy alone. Additionally, those with moderate to severe OCD and those with coexisting mental health conditions such as depression may benefit from the addition of a medication to their treatment regimen.

Medication may also be used temporarily to help an individual cope with the distress induced by the therapy (ERP). Once the individual can cope with the distress on their own, the medication can then be gradually decreased until it is eliminated.

Chapter 7: Cognitive Therapy

Cognitive Therapy, like ERP, is another facet of Cognitive Behavioral Therapy (CBT). CT is typically used in conjunction with ERP in the treatment of OCD. Indeed, evidence shows us that the best results are obtained when people use the two techniques together.

But what exactly is Cognitive Therapy, and how does it differ from Exposure and Response Prevention Therapy?

Identifying Negative Patterns of Thought

The goal of Cognitive Therapy is to help you identify patterns of thought that cause anxiety, distress, and negative behaviors (compulsions). These negative and irrational thoughts are also known as cognitive distortions. Once identified, these distortions can be challenged and replaced with more realistic ways of thinking through a process called cognitive restructuring.

For cognitive restructuring to take place, however, you must first identify your cognitive distortions. This can be particularly tricky, as negative thoughts can come and go in the blink of an eye.

To help you identify your negative thought patterns, we'll review some of the commonly encountered cognitive distortions.

Cognitive Distortions

Magnification and Minimization: In magnification, the importance of a perceived failure, weakness, or threat is exaggerated. In minimization, the importance of a significant event is diminished. An example of minimization might be feeling that a personal achievement such as a good grade in school or an award at work isn't that important compared to "all the mistakes" you've made in your life.

Catastrophizing: Catastrophizing is just like it sounds. When viewing a situation, a person who catastrophizes sees only the worst possible outcome. When thinking about an upcoming job interview, a person who catastrophizes might think, "I'm going to blank out in the middle of the interview or say something stupid. It will probably go so badly that they will cut the interview short, and I won't get the job."

Personalization: This cognitive distortion refers to the belief that one is responsible for events outside of their control. For example, you might observe that your brother has been more down than usual for the last couple of weeks. In response, you might find yourself thinking: "My brother would probably be happier if I were able to spend more time with him."

While you may want your brother to be happy, ultimately, you are not responsible for his happiness, nor can you control his emotional state. Realizing this can be a difficult pill to swallow, but it's necessary to break through the veil of your cognitive distortions.

Overgeneralization: Overgeneralization involves making broad judgments or assumptions based on a single experience or event. The classic example would be assuming that you will never get a job after doing poorly in a job interview.

Fortune Telling: In fortune-telling, the individual predicts that a situation will turn out poorly, without sufficient evidence to support this. An example might be a woman who believes that she will never find love simply because she has not found it yet.

Mind Reading: Similar to fortune telling, mind reading involves making assumptions about the thoughts and beliefs of others, again without adequate evidence. An example might be assuming that your significant other doesn't care about you anymore because they didn't respond to a text message you sent a few hours ago.

Emotional Reasoning: Emotional reasoning is the belief that your emotions reflect the ways things are. For example, you might feel guilty about something; therefore, you conclude that you must be guilty, even without any evidence to support this.

Disqualifying the Positive: This cognitive distortion involves acknowledging the negative aspects of a situation while ignoring the positive. Upon receiving a critique, for example, you might receive mostly positive comments and one negative one. When viewing the critique through this distortion, all you would see would be the one negative comment. None of the positive comments would matter.

All-or-Nothing Thinking: All-or-nothing thinking is just that; your mind thinks in terms of absolutes such as "always," "never," etc. With all or nothing thinking, you might think, "I'll always be a failure," or "I'll never be good at anything."

Now that we've covered some of the most common cognitive distortions, it's time for you to identify your negative patterns of thought. To do this, we have included a "thought record." Thought records are useful tools and can help you identify the thoughts, feelings, and behaviors that accompany an experience. By logging your experiences and the thoughts and feelings that come with them, you will learn to identify your cognitive distortions. Once recognized, you can then begin to challenge these faulty beliefs and replace them with healthier ways of thinking.

Take a moment to review the worksheet below. Once you've finished, you're ready to move on to the next step!

Event	Thought	Feeling	Behavior	Rational Counterstatement
Example: My friend is very upset.	I must have done something wrong.	Thinking about it makes me very anxious and sad.	I was spending large amounts of time obsessing over what I might have done wrong.	There are lots of reasons why my friend could be upset. We get along very well most of the time, so it's unlikely that she's upset at me.

Changing the Way You Think

Once your negative patterns of thought are identified, it's time to challenge them. To help you in this process, we'll cover three cognitive restructuring techniques that you can use to nip your cognitive distortions in the bud and replace them with healthier ways of thinking.

These techniques should be used whenever a cognitive distortion is identified. By repeating this process, your distortions should gradually resolve over time and be replaced by new, rational ways of thinking.

Before we begin, it's worth mentioning two common misconceptions about cognitive restructuring. The first is the belief that cognitive restructuring is simply "positive thinking." This is untrue. Remember, the goal of cognitive restructuring is to think more rationally, not more positively.

The second misconception is the idea that cognitive restructuring is too "simple" to be effective. How can changing the words you use and the way you think impact what you feel and what you do?

The answer is that while cognitive restructuring may seem "simple" at first, it is highly effective in the treatment of OCD. To illustrate this, consider the following example. If you surround yourself with negative people who constantly criticize you and put you down, how are you most likely to react? Even if you know that what the other people are saying isn't true, at some point all of the negative comments are going to get to you.

You may even start to believe that some of them are true. Conversely, if you surround yourself with positive people who support you and care for you, you are more likely to feel happy.

Imagine, therefore, the impact that your negative thoughts have on you over time. By replacing these thoughts with realistic ones, cognitive restructuring encourages healthier thought patterns and can improve the quality of your life.

With that being said, let's discuss the three techniques we mentioned previously. For each method, a worksheet will be provided. Think of these as "homework" assignments in a sense. Each worksheet will help guide you through the process of applying the technique to your everyday life.

Socratic Questioning

Socratic questioning gets its name from the educational method often used by Socrates, the Greek philosopher. The technique emphasizes the importance of exploring thoughts and beliefs by asking questions.

Once a cognitive distortion is identified, the process is relatively straightforward. You will ask yourself a series of questions, such as those provided in the worksheet below. Be sure to take your time when answering the questions. Explore your thoughts and feelings in depth. Scrutinize the evidence. Ideally, you should try to spend at least 1 to 3 minutes on each question.

Through Socratic questioning, you will become more aware of your irrational thoughts and learn to challenge your cognitive distortions.

Socratic Questioning Worksheet Example

Thoughts are powerful things. They can shape the way we feel and even determine how we act. When thoughts become negative or harmful, it's important to challenge them and replace them with healthier thinking patterns.

Take a moment to answer each of the questions below. Try to spend at least 1 to 3 minutes considering each question (or longer if necessary) and be thoughtful in your responses.

Thought to be questioned:

If I touch a public door handle without washing my hands right away, I know I'll get sick.

Is there any evidence to support this thought? What is the evidence against it?

Evidence in support of thought: Lots of people touch public door handles every day. Not everyone practices good hand hygiene, and even those that do might be harboring potentially harmful germs on their hands.

Evidence against thought: While it's true that the door handle may contain harmful germs, the odds of me getting sick from touching it are very small.

Are these thoughts based on facts or feelings?

These thoughts are mainly based on feelings. The idea of coming into contact with germs and getting sick makes me scared.

Could I be misinterpreting something?

I could be misinterpreting my odds of actually getting sick from touching the door handle. In reality, the odds of me getting sick are much smaller than my thoughts suggest.

Am I making assumptions or jumping to conclusions?

I guess I am jumping to conclusions a little bit. My thought is based on the assumption that the door handle contains harmful germs that will make me sick if I touch it and don't wash my hands right away. My odds of actually getting sick from touching the door handle, however, are quite small.

Would other people interpret this situation differently? If so, how would they interpret it?

Other people probably wouldn't be as concerned about touching the door handle. They would probably think that their odds of getting sick from touching the handle are so minuscule that they wouldn't worry too much about it.

Am I considering all the evidence, or am I only looking at the evidence that supports my thought?

I suppose that at first, I was only considering the evidence that supports my thought. For example, I know that the door handle more than likely contains germs, some of which may be harmful. However, I ignored the fact that my odds of becoming sick from touching the door handle are minimal.

Does this thought represent a likely scenario, or am I catastrophizing?

While the scenario of getting sick from touching the door handle isn't impossible, it's doubtful. Looking at it this way, I realize that I am envisioning the worst possible outcome.

Socratic Questioning Worksheet

Thoughts are powerful things. They can shape the way we feel and even determine how we act. When thoughts become negative or harmful, it's important to challenge them and replace them with healthier thinking patterns.

Take a moment to answer each of the questions below. Try to spend at least 1 to 3 minutes considering each question (or longer if necessary) and be thoughtful in your responses.

Thought to be questioned:

Is there any evidence to support this thought? What is the evidence against it?

Are these thoughts based on facts or feelings?

Could I be misinterpreting something?

Am I making assumptions or jumping to conclusions?

Would other people interpret this situation differently? If so, how would they interpret it?

Am I considering all the evidence, or am I only looking at the evidence that supports my thought?

Does this thought represent a likely scenario, or am I catastrophizing?

Putting Thoughts on Trial

In this exercise, you will act as a defense attorney, prosecutor, and judge. The goal is to put your negative thought on "trial" and reach a "verdict" at the end in the form of rational thought. Putting your thoughts on trial can be particularly helpful, as it allows you to view your thoughts from multiple perspectives in a sensible manner.

To start, you will play the role of a defense attorney. At this stage, you will defend your thought and build a case for why you believe the idea to be true. However, there is one caveat. Just like in real life, you can only use verifiable facts in your defense. That means no interpretations, opinions, or guesses!

Afterward, you'll play the part of the prosecutor. For this part of the trial, you will present the evidence you have against your negative thought. Again, you aren't allowed to use interpretations or opinions.

Finally, you will act as the judge. After thoroughly reviewing the evidence for and against your negative thought, you will make a verdict. Remember that the verdict should be in the form of rational thought.

Below you will find a sample "trial" and an additional worksheet where you can put your negative thoughts to the test.

Putting Thoughts on Trial (Sample)

In this exercise, you will be putting your thought on trial. Your job will then be to act as the defense, prosecution, and judge in this process.

As a defense attorney, your job will be to gather evidence in support of your thought. When the time comes to take on the prosecution's role, you must find evidence against your thought. Like a real trial, however, only verifiable facts can be used as evidence. Interpretations, opinions, and guesses are not allowed.

Afterward, you will act as the judge to make a verdict on the case. Remember that the verdict should be based on the evidence and should be in the form of rational thought.

The Thought	The Defense	The Prosecution	The Verdict
My friend probably thinks I'm dumb. (After not knowing the answer to a question they asked.)	I don't always know the answer to questions that I'm asked. ~~I can tell my friend thinks I'm dumb by the way they looked at me.~~ (Not admissible. This is an interpretation.)	I know the answer to most questions that I'm asked. As a student, I always performed well above average and landed a successful career afterward.	As humans, we don't always have the answer to every question, and that's okay. Not knowing the answer to one question does not mean that I am stupid. Knowing this and given my past achievements, there is no evidence to suggest that I am dumb.

83

Putting Thoughts on Trial

In this exercise, you will be putting your thought on trial. Your job will then be to act as the defense, prosecution, and judge in this process.

As a defense attorney, your job will be to gather evidence in support of your thought. When the time comes to take on the prosecution's role, you must find evidence against your thought. Like a real trial, however, only verifiable facts can be used as evidence. Interpretations, opinions, and guesses are not allowed.

Afterward, you will act as the judge to make a verdict on the case. Remember that the verdict should be based on the evidence and should be in the form of rational thought.

The Thought	The Defense	The Prosecution	The Verdict

Decatastrophizing

Decatastrophizing is also known as the "what if" technique and is very straightforward. When confronted with a cognitive distortion, ask yourself simple questions such as "What if?" or "What's the worst thing that could happen?"

An example of decatastrophizing might go something like this:

Thought: I'm always worried when I have to give a presentation at work. I'm so afraid that I'll mess up or say something to make myself look stupid in front of all my co-workers. As a result, I usually get so worked up that I stumble and stammer my way through the presentation.

Question: So, what if you do mess up or say something stupid? What will happen then?

Answer: I'm not sure. I guess I'll feel really anxious and foolish. My co-workers will likely notice my mistake, as well.

Question: What if your co-workers do notice your mistake? What will happen then?

Answer: I don't know. They might think I'm stupid, but more than likely, they'll forget about it in a couple of hours. We've all made mistakes before, and one mistake doesn't necessarily mean my co-workers will think any less of me.

Working your way through this series of questions can help reduce the irrational anxiety associated with your negative thoughts. Additionally, working your way through your "worst-case scenario" can help you realize that even the worst outcome is manageable.

Wrapping Things Up

Changing the way you think isn't something that happens overnight. It's a long and arduous process but well worth the effort in the long run. In fact, studies have shown that more than 85% of people who complete a course of Cognitive Behavioral Therapy experience a significant reduction in their OCD symptoms. However, it should be noted that these statistics come from people who completed an outpatient program under the supervision of a therapist. When attempting CBT on your own, as part of a self-help program, individual results may vary. That doesn't mean that you should let these results deter you. On the contrary, with time and dedication, you may very well experience a reduction in your OCD symptoms and improve your overall quality of life.

Also, be sure to give yourself some downtime and don't spend too long thinking about an exercise or scenario. When you first start, the exercises may take more time as you get used to the techniques. Over time, however, you should be able to move through the activities more quickly. Spending excessive amounts of time agonizing over tiny details isn't helpful and will cause you to burn out fairly quickly. If you feel yourself becoming overwhelmed, don't be afraid to reach out for help! Refer to chapter 16, Getting Help, for additional resources.

Chapter 8: Acceptance and Commitment Therapy

Acceptance and Commitment Therapy (ACT) is part of the so-called "third wave" of Cognitive Behavioral Therapy. It is relatively new as far as treatments go. As a result, there isn't as much evidence for ACT as there is for other forms of CBT (such as ERP, CT, etc.) The evidence that we do have, however, is quite promising and has shown that ACT is an effective treatment for OCD, skin picking, and trichotillomania. Additionally, ACT appears to be well tolerated by those who use it and has a very low drop-out rate compared to ERP. But what is ACT exactly, and how does it differ from ERP?

What is ACT?

Acceptance and Commitment Therapy views obsessions, anxiety, and fear as part of our everyday lives. According to ACT, these thoughts and sensations aren't necessarily bad or harmful. This may seem counterintuitive at first. When experiencing an obsession centered around the fear of contamination, for example, the anxiety and distress that you may encounter are all too real. How could a thought that causes so much fear not be harmful?

According to ACT, it is not the thought itself (the fear of contamination) that is harmful, but our response to that thought (compulsive handwashing.) In essence, while we cannot control our thoughts or feelings, we can control what we do while experiencing these things.

The goal of ACT, therefore, is to allow you to openly experience your obsessions without engaging in your normal compulsive response. In contrast to other forms of CBT, the frequency of your obsessions may remain the same. It is how you allow yourself to experience your obsessions that changes. Ultimately, by the end of therapy, you should be able to experience your obsessive thoughts just as you would any other thought. Through ACT, you will learn to let these thoughts come and go without engaging in your compulsive behaviors. Your obsessions will still be present but won't interfere with your ability to live your life the way you would like to.

The Six Central Processes of ACT

Acceptance and Commitment Therapy revolves around six central processes: acceptance, cognitive diffusion, being present/mindfulness, self as context, values clarification and committed action.

Acceptance: Rather than avoiding or suppressing your thoughts, emotions, and impulses, acceptance encourages you to make space for them in your mind. In doing so, acceptance helps prevent you from over-inflating your thoughts so that you can move on more quickly.

Cognitive diffusion: Cognitive diffusion refers to the process of viewing your psychological experiences objectively. For example, feelings are viewed merely as feelings and don't necessarily indicate that something terrible is about to happen. Similarly, thoughts are just thoughts and aren't necessarily valid or important.

Being present: Being present is also sometimes referred to as mindfulness. It encourages us to immerse ourselves in the present moment. Rather than dwelling on the past or worrying about the future, mindfulness prompts us to take note of how we're currently feeling (mentally and physically) and to completely engage ourselves in the here-and-now.

Self as context: Self as context is sometimes referred to as the observing self and is the process of viewing your psychological and physical experiences as ever-changing processes.

Values clarification: Values clarification is the process of identifying and exploring the things that you believe to be meaningful. Self-reflection exercises that focus on this process can be particularly beneficial in helping you find direction and motivation.

Committed action: Committed action revolves around the process of goal-setting. Acceptance and Commitment Therapy is then used to help you work towards your value-based goals through action.

Is ACT More Effective Than ERP?

As previously mentioned, ACT is a relatively new therapy, and the evidence we have for it is limited compared to other forms of CBT. As such, most experts suggest that ERP used alone or in conjunction with CT should be considered the first line of therapy in the treatment of OCD. However, ACT may be helpful when used in conjunction with ERP, especially for those who are struggling with exposure therapy. ACT may also prove beneficial for people who have had little success with other treatments for their OCD.

ACT Interventions

There are a multitude of ACT interventions available for the treatment of OCD. This is particularly useful as it allows you to experiment with each of the techniques to find the ones that work best for you. Typically, an intervention will focus on one or more of the six key processes listed above. The interventions themselves can last anywhere from a few minutes to more lengthy interventions that span multiple self-guided sessions.

Given the sheer number of cognitive diffusion and mindfulness exercises, we will discuss these subjects in greater detail in subsequent chapters. The following interventions, therefore, will focus on the remaining four key processes of ACT.

Increasing Awareness of Cognitive Distortions

For this exercise, we'll be taking another look at cognitive distortions, albeit from a slightly different perspective. While traditional CBT focuses on restructuring your cognitive distortions, ACT focuses on making room for these thoughts and accepting them for what they are.

To make room for these distortions in your mind, however, you must first learn to identify them. This exercise will focus on helping you identify your cognitive distortions and the feelings associated with them.

Start by identifying what you are feeling in the present moment. Are you afraid of something? Anxious? Sad? What physical sensations do you have? For example, do you feel tense? Are you tired?

Next, identify the thoughts running through your mind when these feelings and sensations occur. Consider for a moment how your thoughts and emotions relate to one another.

Finally, identify the cognitive distortion that might be at work.

To aid in the exercise, we have created a worksheet where you can jot down your thoughts and feelings and the cognitive distortion they represent.

Increasing Awareness of Cognitive Distortions Worksheet

Feelings and Physical Sensations	Thoughts	Cognitive Distortion
Example: I feel incredibly anxious. My body feels jittery, and I can feel my heart racing in my chest.	*Example: I know I'm going to fail this exam.*	*Example: Catastrophizing (Assuming the worst possible outcome of an event.)*

Identifying Emotional Avoidance Strategies

Avoidance is a common strategy people employ when confronted with uncomfortable thoughts and feelings. And while avoidance may seem helpful in the short-term, it is ultimately ineffective in helping you cope with your thoughts and feelings over time. In fact, avoidance only serves to reinforce and intensify your negative thoughts and emotions.

In this exercise, you will learn to identify when you are trying to escape from unwanted thoughts, feelings, or memories. This information can then be used to identify common tactics or habits you routinely use to avoid dealing with these unwanted thoughts and feelings emotionally.

To start the exercise, recall a time when you actively avoided an uncomfortable thought, feeling, or memory rather than engaging with it.

Ask yourself the following questions:

What feelings did I experience?

What did I do to avoid those unwanted thoughts or feelings? Did I do something mentally to avoid those things? Did I engage in a specific behavior?

How useful was the avoidance strategy that I used?

After completing the exercise, review your responses. Do you notice any patterns in your behavior? For example, when confronted with uncomfortable thoughts of contamination, do you engage in excessive handwashing? Or do you avoid touching "contaminated" objects altogether?

Once you identify your emotional avoidance strategies, consider alternative behaviors or approaches that you could have adopted instead. Would these alternative strategies have produced different results?

To facilitate this exercise, we have included a worksheet that you can use as you work your way through the questions.

Identifying Emotional Avoidance Strategies Worksheet

1. Recall a time when you actively avoided an uncomfortable thought, feeling, or memory rather than engaging with it. What was the thought or feeling that you were trying to avoid?

2. What feelings did you experience? For example, were you anxious? Did you feel embarrassed or sad?

3. What did you do to avoid these unwanted thoughts or emotions? Did you do something mentally, such as trying to suppress the negative

thought? Or did you engage in a particular behavior?

4. How useful was this avoidance strategy?

5. When reviewing your avoidance strategies, do you notice any patterns? If so, what are they?

6. What alternative behaviors or approaches could you have used instead? Could these alternative strategies have produced different results?

Ball in a Pool: An Expansion and Acceptance Metaphor

ACT often makes use of metaphors to help us understand the impact our thoughts and emotions have on our behaviors while simultaneously allowing us to reconceptualize these processes in more adaptive ways. One such metaphor is that of a ball in a pool.

For this exercise, let your thoughts and emotions take the shape of a beachball in a pool.

You want to enjoy your time in the water; however, you find that you are unable to do so as the beachball keeps floating and bumping into you. Desperately, you want the beachball to go away, so you try and submerge it in the water. Inevitably, once you let go, the beachball bounces back to the surface and continues to bother you. Only by repeatedly forcing the beachball underwater and holding it there can you keep it submerged. However, this process takes effort, and to keep the beachball submerged, you must also keep it close to you.

What, then, is the solution to this problem? The answer is to let the beachball go. This may cause discomfort at first, but eventually, the beachball will drift away from you. The ball will still be there, floating elsewhere in the pool, but it won't prevent you from enjoying your time in the water anymore.

As this exercise illustrates, only by acknowledging and accepting our thoughts can we truly break free from them. The thoughts and feelings are still there, but we adapt and learn to live with them.

Emotional Acceptance: Observing Your Emotions

This exercise is adapted from a workbook called "Get Out of Your Mind and Into Your Life" by Dr. Steven Hayes. The exercise should be done when you are experiencing an uncomfortable emotion. The emotion should be strong enough for you to recognize its presence but not so strong that you find yourself completely overwhelmed by it.

Begin the exercise by identifying the emotion. If you find yourself experiencing multiple emotions, pick one to focus on. You can always come back to the other emotions later. Once you have identified the feeling, write it down on a piece of paper.

Next, close your eyes. Picture the emotion standing several feet away from you in your mind. When looking at your emotion, how would you describe it? If your emotion had a size, what size would it be? What color would it be? Does it have a shape?

Once you are done characterizing your emotion, envision it in front of you using the size, shape, and color that you gave it. Observe your emotion. Recognize it for what it is without judgment. When you feel you are ready, let the emotion return to its original place inside of you.

Once you have completed the exercise, it's time to reflect on your experience. Ask yourself the following questions:

Did you notice any change in the way you perceived your emotion once you were able to distance yourself from it?

Did you react any differently to the emotion?

How did you describe your emotion? What size, color, and shape did you give it?

Once the exercise was over, did the emotion feel different in any way?

This exercise may seem a little odd at first, but we encourage you to give it a try. Over time the exercise will help change the way you think about your emotions and will help you become more accepting of them.

Not This, Not That Exercise

This exercise was originally presented by Russ Harris at the 2009 ACT World Conference. It's a short exercise that can be completed in a few minutes and emphasizes the self as context process of ACT.

Start by focusing your attention on your breathing. Allow yourself to observe the flow of your breath as you breathe in and out. As you do this, acknowledge the fact that you are merely an observer. Therefore, if you can observe your breath, you cannot be your breath.

As you move through the exercise, notice how your breathing changes over time. Your breath, by its very nature, is constantly changing. As an observer, however, you remain separate from your breath and do not change.

Once you have completed the exercise, consider how your breathing (in the context of this exercise) relates to your thoughts and feelings. Like your breathing, your thoughts and emotions are continuous and constantly changing.

Values

As you move through the exercises in this workbook, it may be helpful to explore and reflect upon your values. Identifying your values can help you set life goals and can be a helpful reminder of why you are doing this when the going gets tough.

For this exercise, you will be given a list of ten categories. For each category, consider what values, goals, etc. are most important to you (Wilson and Murrell, 2004). Each category contains sample questions that you may wish to ask yourself as you consider your goals. As you move through the exercise, we encourage you to create your own questions to further clarify your goals in each category.

Below, you will find the Values worksheet with sample questions.

Values Worksheet

1. Romantic relationships: If you could create an ideal relationship, what would it be like? What sort of partner do you aspire to be?

2. Leisure and fun: What kinds of activities do you do for fun? When you have some time to relax and unwind, what do you like to do? What do you consider to be relaxing? Conversely, what do you find to be exciting?

3. Job/Career: What are your career goals? What kind of employment appeals to you? Are there any qualities as a worker that you aspire to?

4. Friends: What kinds of social relationships do you consider to be important? How would you like to develop these relationships? What would you like your friends to think of you as a person?

5. Health and wellness: How would you describe your idea of what it means to be healthy (both physically and mentally)? How important is your health and wellbeing to you? How about personal care? What are your fitness goals?

6. Parenthood: What kind of mother or father would you like to be? What would you like your relationship with your children to be like? Additionally, what sort of role-model would you like to be?

7. Social citizenship: What role would you like to play in your community? How would you like your community to see you as a person?

8. Family relationships: This category is similar to parenthood (above) and pertains to other family members such as parents, siblings, extended family, etc.

9. Spirituality: Questions in this section may concern religion or anything meaningful at a deeper level. For example, consider your moral code. How would you describe it? Are your beliefs based upon the teachings of a particular religion or from some other source?

10. Personal development and growth: Are you knowledgeable in any particular field? What are

your capabilities, competencies, and skills? How would you like to grow and develop your skills and knowledge? How would you like to change as a person?

Commitment, Obstacles, and Strategies

Just as the name suggests, this exercise is all about maintaining your motivation and resolution as you pursue your goals.

Drawing from the values you identified in the previous exercise, identify a commitment that you'd like to make. Next, consider potential obstacles that you may encounter as you work towards your commitment. Afterward, try to think of ways you could address or work around these obstacles.

Complete this for as many commitments you would like to make. However, remember to keep your commitments reasonable and not to stretch yourself too thin. Below you will find a worksheet that you may wish to use as a guide as you work through this exercise.

Commitment, Obstacles and Strategies Worksheet

Commitment	Potential Obstacles	Strategies for Boosting Commitment
Example: I want to spend more time being social with my friends.	*I get anxious when I'm around other people (especially if I'm in a public place) and often try to avoid social gatherings.*	*I will create an ERP program that exposes me to public places. ACT exercises such as Identifying Emotional Avoidance Strategies and Emotional Acceptance may also be useful.*

Chapter 9: Cognitive Diffusion and Mindfulness

As we discussed in the previous chapter, both cognitive diffusion and mindfulness are critical aspects of ACT. Given the sheer number of cognitive diffusion and mindfulness exercises, we have dedicated an entire chapter to these subjects.

Cognitive Diffusion

In a sense, our brain can be thought of as a machine. It's primary job, in this sense, is to generate thought afterthought. Most of the thoughts running through our heads tend to be random. Some of these thoughts may even be helpful. However, many thoughts may be negative, harmful, or stem from deep-seated fear.

These thoughts are often hypothetical and may consist of "what if" scenarios and other things or events we don't have control over. But why does our brain do this? After all, if these thoughts truly are negative or harmful, why would our brain continue to focus on them?

Evolutionarily speaking, our ancestors evolved for survival. Over time, the human brain evolved accordingly, becoming disproportionately aware of sources of danger. While this proved useful to the survival of our ancestors (and still is useful in certain situations), it is also the reason we sometimes have difficulty "turning off" these negative thoughts. Your brain does not recognize that what it is doing is harmful – it is merely doing its job. In this case, your brain is trying to make you aware of potential sources of danger, whether the danger is valid or not.

Fortunately, our higher brain structures allow us to reconceptualize these thoughts and how we relate to them. For example, the following thought might occur to you: *"I'm sure that the TV remote is covered with all kinds of harmful bacteria and viruses. If I touch it, I know, I will get sick."* Thinking rationally about it, you recognize that this thought is based on your fear of contamination and does not necessarily represent reality. By acknowledging this thought and letting it pass through your mind without dwelling on it, you can let go of the fear and move on.

Cognitive Fusion

When we over-identify with our thoughts and amplify them, we can enter a state of cognitive fusion. In this state, our thoughts are treated as "facts" or "the truth" regardless of whether they are or not. When this occurs, our thoughts can become overbearing and, in some cases controlling.

Cognitive defusion can be used to help you distance yourself from these thoughts through a variety of techniques. Rather than holding onto the thought or accepting it as the truth, cognitive defusion teaches you to let your thoughts come and go without reflecting on them. It also emphasizes the point that thoughts are just thoughts, nothing more. They are not necessarily true or important.

Before we get into some cognitive defusion techniques, it's worth mentioning that the exercises we will be covering for cognitive defusion and mindfulness are not meant to replace ERP, medications, etc. Rather, they are meant to be helpful tools that you can use to "get yourself out of your head," if only for a few minutes.

External Voice

Pay close attention to your thoughts and the language that you use. For example, instead of thinking, "Someone is going to break into the house if I don't check to see if the door is locked," practice thinking, "My brain is giving me the thought that someone could break into the house if I don't make sure the door is locked."

It's amazing how changing the language we use can impact how we feel and how we relate to our thoughts. This technique also acts as a reminder that our thoughts aren't necessarily true. Just because your brain is telling you that someone is going to break into the house if you don't check that the door is locked does not mean that someone is going to break in.

Passengers on a Bus

In this exercise, imagine that you are a bus driver. Unfortunately for you, there are more than a few rowdy and troublesome passengers aboard your vehicle. Picture your obsessions and negative thoughts as these problem passengers.

Your goal is to remain focused and arrive safely at your destination. During this trip, you must continue driving, despite what your passengers may tell you. This means no stopping along the way (to let a passenger off or forcibly remove them from the bus yourself.)

Will you be able to remain focused and make it to your destination without making any stops?

Say It Slowly/Sing Your Obsessions to a Song

These exercises are fairly straightforward. To complete the first exercise, practice saying your thought in slow motion. Repeat this until the thought begins to lose its power. Is the thought as frightening or uncomfortable as it was before you started the exercise?

Similarly, try singing your thoughts or obsessions to a song. Rinse and repeat until the thought begins to lose its power over you.

Leaves on a Stream

Leaves on a stream is a very well known technique that can be used to create some space between you and your thoughts. When a thought or obsession surfaces in your mind, picture yourself placing it on a leaf. Then, imagine yourself placing the leaf on a gentle stream. Watch the leaf as it is carried by the current and floats away until you lose sight of it in the distance.

Assign a Character to Your Brain's Obsessions

We've saved a bit of a fun one for last. As the name suggests, you will assign a character to your brain's obsessions and negative thoughts. Whenever the thought or obsession pops into your head, it will take the form of the character you chose. According to Dr. Ryan Vidrine, an Interventional Psychiatrist at TMS Health Solutions in San Francisco, something "cheeky and outrageous tends to work best, as humor is one of the best-known defusion techniques."

For example, your thoughts and obsessions centered around your fear of contamination might take on the form of Darth Vader. Additionally, you might imagine your perfection obsessions as characters from a favorite TV show or cartoon.

While this technique might seem a bit absurd, we highly recommend giving it a try. Doing so might allow you to break free from your thoughts, if only for a few minutes. And who knows, you might just have some fun along the way.

Mindfulness

Odds are, you've heard about mindfulness before. In the last few years, the concept has gained quite a bit of popularity as a method of stress reduction and has even been used in the treatment of certain mental illnesses.

Mindfulness can be described as immersing yourself completely in the present moment without judgment. When practicing mindfulness, your focus is on the present, not the past or the future. All physical sensations and thoughts are allowed to come and go, without dwelling on them or judging them in any way. In doing so, mindfulness can help you learn to accept the present moment for what it is and move on.

Thought-Act Fusion

For someone with OCD, mindfulness may seem like a challenging concept. For example, consider all the time someone with OCD spends worrying about whether they did something wrong in the past, or agonizing about what might go wrong in the future.

And what about remaining non-judgemental? Odds are, if you have OCD, you constantly blame yourself for bad things that may have happened in the past or for bad things that might happen in the future. In some cases, individuals may spend hours reviewing past events and what they should have done differently. Similarly, a person may incessantly agonize over what may happen in the future.

One pitfall that many people with OCD fall into is that of thought-act fusion. Thought-act fusion is a type of cognitive distortion in which a person believes that thinking a bad thought is equivalent to performing the action associated with the thought. Additionally, individuals may also believe that simply thinking about certain thoughts can make those thoughts come true.

Take, for example, the case of a new mother. Occasionally, some mothers may experience thoughts of harming their baby. However, these thoughts are not reflective of the way the mother feels about her child, and so, most women recognize these thoughts as being meaningless and can let them go. A mother experiencing thought-act fusion, however, is unable to break free from these thoughts. Immediately, they assume that they must be a terrible person for thinking such a thing. After all, what parent thinks of their child in such a way? Is she even fit to be a parent? Thus, through judgment and self-criticism, these negative thoughts are allowed to continue unabated.

How is Mindfulness Used to Treat OCD?

In a sense, mindfulness is similar to ERP. Looking back to chapter 5, recall that ERP required you to intentionally expose yourself to a trigger while simultaneously resisting the urge to give in to your compulsive response. Similarly, in mindfulness, you are also exposed to a trigger (whether intentional or not) however; mindfulness differs from ERP in how you are tasked with perceiving and responding to a trigger.

When practicing mindfulness, your objective is to simply remain aware that you have encountered a trigger. Once you become aware of a trigger, mindfulness teaches you to accept the trigger, along with the discomfort it causes. When observing your trigger, you must do so without judgment and without trying to suppress it in any way. Allow yourself to experience your trigger, however uncomfortable it might be. As you do this, resist the urge to give in to your compulsive responses.

By utilizing mindfulness, you will learn to accept thoughts simply as mental events. While you can observe these thoughts, they are not necessarily harmful or indicative that something terrible is going to happen.

Practicing Mindfulness

The practice of mindfulness can take on many forms. For example, practicing mindfulness can be as simple as remaining aware of what is going on within and around you over the course of your day. Next time you are brushing your teeth, pay attention to the flavor of your toothpaste. You would be surprised at the number of people who realize that they can't stand the taste of their toothpaste once they truly allow themselves to experience the act of brushing their teeth.

Mindfulness can take on other forms as well, such as mindfulness meditation, visualization, and mindful movement, which will be discussed in further detail below.

Mindfulness Meditation

Meditation is one of the most widely recognized forms of mindfulness. Depending on your preferences, mindfulness meditation can be carried out on your own or through guided meditation.

When using guided meditation, another person guides you step-by-step through the meditation process. This can be done in person, through a video, app, etc. Given the vast number of videos and apps featuring guided meditation, we will refrain from covering them in this book and instead focus on solo meditation.

Solo meditation, as the name implies, is carried out on your own. Before starting a meditation session, make sure that you have enough time set aside (around 10 to 15 minutes should be sufficient).

The next step can be a little tricky, depending on your living situation, as it entails finding a quiet, calm space where you won't be interrupted. Once you have a place picked out, find a comfortable spot to sit or lie down in. For the purposes of the exercise, your body position does not matter as long as you are comfortable.

While in this position, allow yourself to relax completely. Then, focus your attention on your breathing. Draw your attention to each breath as you breathe in and back out again. Allow your thoughts to come and go as you do this. Don't dwell on these thoughts. Merely observe them and accept them for what they are, without judgment. If your mind begins to wander, gently bring it back to the present moment.

Ultimately, the goal of this exercise is for you to reach a state of relaxation and mindfulness.

Visualization

Visualization is typically a guided process. As with guided meditation, the session may be carried out by a guide in person or through a video, audio file, or app. For this reason, it is often referred to as guided imagery or guided visualization. Before starting the exercise, your guide will transition you into a relaxed, meditative state. Afterward, you will be guided through various scenes, in which you will use all of your senses to make the scene as vivid as possible.

The primary focus of visualization will depend upon your goal for the session. For example, visualization can be used simply as a relaxation technique or to help address anxiety or intrusive thoughts. When used in the treatment of OCD, your goals may differ slightly. In this case, your goal might be to overcome your fears or to prepare yourself for a triggering situation. Recall imaginal exposure from chapter 5. To prepare yourself for a trigger in real life, imaginal exposure had you confront the trigger in your mind first. While you may not have realized it at first, this was visualization in action.

Other goals of visualization might include imagining what your life would be like if you were able to break free from your OCD symptoms or visualizing yourself, taking back control of your life.

Additionally, the Liquid Quiet Technique can be used to help focus your thoughts when you feel your mind racing. Before starting, you may wish to find a quiet, comfortable space where you are less likely to be disturbed. Next, visualize 'quiet' in your mind. Allow it to take the form of a thick, clear liquid that fills your head with peace and quiet. Visualize the liquid as it flows slowly down your body until you are completely covered by this soothing, liquid ball. Once you have achieved this state of calm relaxation, take several deep breaths, and remain in this position for a few more minutes.

Mindful Movement

Mindful movement utilizes slow, flowing movements such as those found in Yoga, tai chi, and pilates. As you go through these motions, you will be tasked with focusing your mind entirely on the present moment. For example, you could focus on the movements of your body. What do they feel like? How do you feel while you are performing them?

Mindfulness meditation isn't limited to the exercises listed above. Any exercise can become mindful – so long as you commit yourself to focus entirely on the present moment as you do so.

Let's say you fancy a swim and decide to take a few laps around your pool. What does the water feel like on your skin? Is it cold? Luke-warm? What does it feel like as your body moves through the water?

The possibilities are endless when it comes to mindful movement. Additionally, those who have difficulty sitting or lying still when practicing mindfulness might find this technique helpful. Plus, it allows you to work some exercise into your schedule at the same time (along with all of the health benefits that exercise provides)! It's a win-win.

Can Mindfulness Weaken the Effectiveness of ERP?

Over the years, mindfulness has proven to be an effective tool in the treatment of certain mental health conditions, including OCD. Despite these promising results, however, there is some concern that mindfulness strategies, when used incorrectly, can weaken the effectiveness of ERP. This does not mean that mindfulness strategies should not be used, but that care should be taken to use them correctly.

This begs the question – at what point does mindfulness cross the threshold from helpful to harmful?

Mindfulness is centered around the concept of accepting your thoughts, physical sensations, etc., in the present moment for what they are and nothing more. It's when this concept becomes a mantra, so to speak, that mindfulness becomes harmful to your recovery process. The mantra, when used in this way, becomes a way to reassure yourself that your fears will not come true. In doing so, you prevent yourself from confronting your fears. And when you don't confront your fears, you cannot hope to overcome them.

When used in conjunction with ERP, practicing mindfulness incorrectly can be particularly harmful. Recall that for ERP to be effective you must expose yourself to a trigger and the fear and discomfort that comes along with it. If you don't allow yourself to experience your fear (and reap the benefits of habituation over time), the ERP is rendered useless.

However, don't let this deter you from using mindfulness techniques altogether. In particular, mindfulness has shown promise in the treatment of OCD when used in conjunction with CBT. In fact, mindfulness may even enhance the effectiveness of CBT.

For example, when used in conjunction with ERP, mindfulness can be used to help you acknowledge and accept the uncomfortable reactions you may have towards a trigger. By openly allowing yourself to experience your fear and discomfort, you reduce the power your compulsions have over you and enhance the effectiveness of ERP.

Chapter 10: Relaxation Techniques

Stress and OCD

As we already know, stress is a potent trigger for OCD. As such, it's not uncommon for people with the condition to report an increase in the number or severity of their stressors just before their symptoms worsen. But what exactly is stress and why do people react to it differently?

Defining Stress

While we've all experienced a stressful event in our lives, defining stress can be a tricky business. The reason for this is that stress can mean different things to different people. For example, one person might consider getting up and singing in front of a large crowd of people to be a stressful event. To a seasoned vocalist, however, this event may be minimally stressful or not stressful at all.

Therefore, when trying to understand the concept of stress, it may be helpful to look at stress from three different perspectives:

Stress as an Event: In this context, stress can be thought of as an event that exceeds our ability to cope.

125

The event, in this situation, is often referred to as a stressor. Stressors may constitute significant life events such as losing your job, getting a divorce, or being diagnosed with a serious illness. Conversely, stressors can be something small, such as the little hassles we face every day. Consider a time when you forgot something on your shopping list, for example. While this may seem small, perhaps even insignificant to some, to others, the stress of forgetting the item (and having to run back to the store) is very real. While stressors will vary from person to person, it's generally believed that the more long-standing, unpredictable, and uncontrollable you perceive a stressor to be, the greater the impact it will have on you.

Stress as a Reaction: Think of this as the classic "fight or flight response." When confronted with an acute stressor (anything that you perceive to be mentally or physically frightening), your body activates a series of physiological and behavioral pathways to help you respond to this perceived threat. The ensuing release of hormones known as catecholamines (such as adrenaline and noradrenaline), activation of stress-sensitive brain regions, and physical responses (such as dilated pupils, increase in blood pressure, rapid heart rate, and breathing) are all designed to keep you alive when confronted with a dangerous situation. In this respect, the "fight or flight" response is your body's way of warning you that something is wrong.

In the short-term, your body's stress response isn't necessarily a bad thing – in some situations, it may even be beneficial. For example, your body's stress response can help enhance your performance in a situation where you are under a lot of pressure, such as school or work. When confronted with a life-threatening situation, the "fight or flight" response is critical to your survival.

However, our "fight or flight" response isn't always accurate. In some cases, our stress response can become triggered, even when there is no real threat. A classic example of this would be phobias.

Additionally, our bodies are not designed to deal with prolonged stress. Over time, the stress response takes a toll on both our bodies and minds and can contribute to the development of depression, anxiety, cardiovascular disease, and diabetes. In individuals with OCD, stress can create a particularly vicious cycle in which external stressors and the stress related to the disorder feed off of each other.

Learning to recognize your body's "fight or flight" response can help you learn to cope with stressful situations.

Stress as a Transaction: Rather than viewing stress as an event or reaction, this concept views stress as a transaction between you and your environment. For example, consider all of the demands that are constantly being placed upon you. Whether you're tasked with paying bills, taking care of a loved one, or fighting traffic to get to work on time, the list of demands can seem endless. To meet these demands, you are expected to provide a variety of resources such as time, knowledge, money, social support, etc. In this context, stress occurs when you believe that you don't have the necessary resources to meet all of the demands placed upon you.

One interesting feature of this model (compared to the previous ones), is that it may explain why people handle stressful situations differently. After all, not everyone views the demands placed upon them or their capacity to deal with those demands in the same way.

Relaxation Techniques

Now that we have reviewed stress and it's link with OCD in further detail, it's time to move on to some helpful relaxation techniques. As with cognitive defusion and mindfulness, these techniques are not meant to replace traditional ERP. Rather, they are meant to be an additional tool you can pull out when you need to unwind and reduce your stress levels.

The exercises below are adapted from Owen Kelly, Ph.D.'s "Relaxation Techniques for OCD" (as medically reviewed by Steven Gans, MD).

Deep Breathing Exercises

Deep breathing, or "diaphragmatic breathing," as it is also known, is an incredibly potent relaxation technique. When you engage in diaphragmatic breathing, strong relaxation signals are sent to your brain. In response, your body begins to relax, resulting in a decrease in your blood pressure, heart rate, and breathing. This, in turn, results in a reduction in stress levels as well.

Before starting the deep breathing exercise, locate a quiet room where you are unlikely to be disturbed. Find a comfortable position, either sitting or lying down – again, the position itself does not matter as long as you are comfortable. Next, place one hand on your chest and the other hand over your stomach. If you feel comfortable, close your eyes.

Start by taking a deep breath in through your nose. As you breathe in, you should feel the hand on your stomach move outward as your stomach expands. At the same time, the hand over your chest should remain almost motionless. This is how you know whether you are performing the technique correctly or not.

Once you are done breathing in, exhale slowly through pursed lips (think of the face you might make if you were trying to whistle). You should feel the hand on your stomach begin to move inwards, towards your spine. Again, the hand over your chest should remain almost motionless. The entire process of exhalation should take about two to three times as long as inhalation.
To get the best results, deep breathing sessions should run anywhere from 5 to 20 minutes.

Progressive Muscle Relaxation

Progressive muscle relaxation can be performed on your own or as a guided exercise. Generally, it involves tensing certain areas of your body as you inhale and relaxing those same areas as you exhale. Occasionally, progressive muscle relaxation is combined with visualization or deep breathing.

In addition to helping with anxiety, progressive muscle relaxation has also been shown to help reduce the muscle tension that often accompanies this condition. Progressive muscle relaxation can also be a helpful tool for those that have difficulty falling asleep at night. When used for this purpose, perform the exercise as you lay in a comfortable position in your bed.

As with deep breathing, start by finding a comfortable position in a quiet location. Again, whether you choose to sit or lay down does not matter – all that matters is that you are comfortable.

Begin the exercise by clenching all of the muscles in your face as you inhale. Hold this position for 10 to 20 seconds, then slowly exhale. As you breathe out, gradually release all of the tension in your muscles. Repeat this an additional 1 to 2 times before moving on to the next body region. As you progress through the exercise, move down your body. Focus your efforts on your shoulders, followed by your arms, forearms, hands, stomach, buttocks, legs, calves, and then feet. As you move through each body region, repeat the process of inhalation/tensing and exhalation/relaxing.

Chapter 11: Hyper-responsibility

Defining Hyper-responsibility

It is completely natural, as humans, to feel a sense of responsibility for the welfare of others. For example, consider a mother's concern for the health and safety of her child. Or the charitable efforts of organizations such as Feeding America, the Salvation Army, and the American Red Cross. In this context, the drive to take care of others generally results in favorable outcomes for both parties. When this sense of responsibility is blown out of proportion, however, it can have negative implications.

Hyper-responsibility is also known as the "savior complex," and for a good reason. Rather than believing themselves to be partially responsible for the health, safety, and wellbeing of others, people with hyper-responsibility believe that they are completely responsible. Often, this is to the detriment of their wellbeing as these individuals neglect their own needs to ensure the happiness of others.

For those with hyper-responsibility, it can feel like the weight of the world is on your shoulders at times. It's not uncommon to feel like only you can solve the problems of the world. And if something bad happens, that you alone are to blame.

The Many Forms of Hyper-responsibility

Conversations/Social Interactions: For those with OCD, this exaggerated sense of responsibility can take on many forms. Even something as mundane as an everyday conversation or a brief interaction with another person can become a minefield of fear and doubt. For example, after talking with a friend, a person with hyper-responsibility might review the conversation over and over again to ensure that nothing offensive or insulting was said. Their fear may even drive them to seek reassurance from their friend that they were not offended by the conversation in any way. As with other compulsive behaviors, the reassurance provided is temporary. Ultimately, the fear resurfaces again, resulting in a continuous cycle of obsessive thoughts and anxiety-relieving behaviors that can place strain on relationships.

Contamination/Environmental Hazards: When individuals with hyper-responsibility suffer from contamination phobias, their main concern is causing the illness or death of others rather than themselves. As a result, they may engage in compulsive cleaning rituals or constantly survey the environment for potential hazards. Cooking for others can also become an impossible task, as these individuals may meticulously check the food repeatedly to make sure that it is cooked properly and is free from contaminants such as cleaners, poisons, germs, etc.

Some individuals may even take it upon themselves to remain hypervigilant of their surroundings. If a potential hazard is identified, they believe that it is their duty to either report the hazard or fix it themselves. For example, if a person with hyper-responsibility OCD noticed that a traffic light wasn't working, they would feel obligated to report it to the relevant authorities. Failure to do so (especially if an accident were to occur as a result of the light being out) would cause significant anxiety, guilt, and shame.

Hit-And-Run OCD: Another example of hyper-responsibility is known as "hit-and-run OCD." Recall our example from chapter 2 of the man who was terrified of accidentally running over someone with his car. For these individuals, even a small bump in the road may be enough to trigger the fear that they may have run over someone. To reassure themselves that this is not the case, they may circle back and drive the route repeatedly, checking frantically for potential victims or emergency vehicles.

Isolation: It's not uncommon for those with hyper-responsibility OCD to isolate themselves from their family and friends. This is not because they don't care or don't want to be around them. Rather, the thought of hurting their loved ones is so distressing, they believe that self-isolating is the best way to protect them.

Donating Money: In an attempt to "fix" individual or world problems, others may donate significant amounts of money to charities or other people. While donating money to a worthy cause can be a noble gesture, individuals with hyper-responsibility take this to the extreme. Often, this results in financial strain or ruin, leaving individuals with insufficient funds to pay bills or see to their personal needs.

How is it Treated?

CBT is the preferred method of treatment for this type of OCD and is often broken down into two phases. First,

ERP is used to help address the anxiety associated with certain thoughts and scenarios. After the individual has dealt with their anxiety, they are ready to challenge their faulty beliefs using CT.

As we have already discussed ERP and CT in previous chapters, we won't be discussing them in detail here. For a complete review of both ERP and CT, it may be helpful to briefly review chapters 5 and 7 of this book before moving on.

The remainder of this chapter will be geared towards helping you build your own ERP plan. Once you have completed your ERP plan in its entirety, you will be tasked with utilizing CT techniques to challenge your beliefs and reshape your role in the responsibility of others.

Building Your ERP Plan

The process of creating an ERP plan is much the same as before. For your convenience, we have included the worksheet from chapter 5 (along with a sample plan) on the following pages.

Remember that your ERP sessions should last anywhere from 60 to 90 minutes. To ensure that your sessions are effective, expect to continue the exposure until you experience at least a 50% reduction in your anxiety.

Allow yourself to experience the exposure completely. Acknowledge your discomfort and any physical sensations you may experience. During this time, you must refrain from engaging in your compulsive responses. Doing so will render the therapy obsolete and will only reinforce your obsessive thoughts, feelings, etc. ERP is a gradual process, so it may take time before you notice a change. However, given enough time (and with the help of habituation), you will experience a reduction in your anxiety.

Creating an ERP Plan

The following worksheet can be used as a guide to create a personalized ERP plan. At the end of the worksheet, you will find a chart to document your progress over time. Remember that this is a gradual process, so don't get discouraged if you don't notice an improvement in your symptoms right away!

Step 1: Setting Realistic Goals

Make a list of your obsessions. Start with the obsession that is the least distressing and work your way up to the most uncomfortable. Ranking each obsession using a 0 – 10 numeric scale may be helpful. Take note of your list, as this is the order you will be completing them in.

Step 2: Imaginal Exposure/Exposure Therapy

Visualize the trigger in your mind to start. Writing the content of your obsession down or making an audio recording of yourself may also be helpful. When you feel you are ready, move on to confronting the trigger in real life. Pay close attention to what you are feeling, both emotionally and physically.

What feelings are you experiencing?

Are you experiencing any physical symptoms?

Step 3: Response Prevention

Refrain from giving in to your compulsive thoughts and behaviors. Don't try to distract yourself or avoid facing the trigger. Acknowledge both the trigger and the feelings and sensations that come with it. Remember, the short term discomfort is well worth the long term gain of being freed from the cycle of your obsessions and compulsions! Don't seek reassurance either, as reassurance interferes with the recovery process. Continue the session until you experience at least a 50% reduction in your symptoms.

Step 4: Keep With It!

Try to be consistent with your sessions. Remember that sessions may take 60 minutes or longer, especially when first starting. Over time, you should notice a gradual decrease in your symptoms. By the end of treatment, the same triggers that were so distressing before should evoke little to no response.

Step 5: You Did It!

Congratulations, you made it! All that hard work has finally paid off, and you are one step closer to freeing yourself from the cycle of your obsessions and compulsions. With one obsession out of the way, it's time to move on to the next one.

Sample ERP Plan

Name Cindy S.

Step 1: Setting Realistic Goals

Make a list of your obsessions. Start with the obsession that is the least distressing and work your way up to the most uncomfortable. Ranking each obsession using a 0 – 10 numeric scale may be helpful. Take note of your list, as this is the order you will be completing them in.

I am so afraid of causing the serious illness or death of someone from my cooking, either by failing to cook the food properly or by accidentally contaminating the food with a harmful substance. As a result, it often takes me hours to prepare even a simple meal for my family and friends.

My level of discomfort is 6-8/10.

Step 2: Imaginal Exposure/Exposure Therapy

Visualize the trigger in your mind to start. Writing the content of your obsession down or making an audio recording of yourself may also be helpful. When you feel you are ready, move on to confronting the trigger in real life. Pay close attention to what you are feeling, both emotionally and physically.

Exposure Therapy: I will invite family and friends over for dinner 3 to 5 times a week.

What feelings are you experiencing?

I feel extremely anxious. I'm worried I may seriously harm or kill a loved one through some carelessness or negligence on my part. I'm afraid that if I don't cook the meat properly, they may get sick from salmonella or some other harmful bacteria.

I also sanitize my countertops regularly using a cleaner that is harmful if ingested. I worry that somehow the food may become contaminated by some residual cleaner on this surface.

Are you experiencing any physical symptoms?

I feel a tightness in my chest, and my hands feel cold and clammy.

Step 3: Response Prevention

Refrain from giving in to your compulsive thoughts and behaviors. Don't try to distract yourself or avoid facing the trigger. Acknowledge both the trigger and the feelings and sensations that come with it. Remember, the short term discomfort is well worth the long term gain of being freed from the cycle of your obsessions and compulsions! Don't seek reassurance either, as reassurance interferes with the recovery process. Continue the session until you experience at least a 50% reduction in your symptoms.

When preparing the meal, I won't stop to inspect, smell, or taste the food for signs of contamination. Once I have finished preparing the food, I will serve it directly to my family/friends without examining it beforehand.

After the meal, I won't call my family or friends to reassure myself that they are okay.

Step 4: Keep With It!

Try to be consistent with your sessions. Remember that sessions may take 60 minutes or longer, especially when first starting. Over time, you should notice a gradual decrease in your symptoms. By the end of treatment, the same triggers that were so distressing before should evoke little to no response.

Over the past few weeks, I have noticed a steady decline in my symptoms. Initially, I was experiencing 6-8/10 discomfort. Now, however, my level of discomfort has decreased to 2/10.

Step 5: You Did It!

Congratulations, you made it! All that hard work has finally paid off, and you are one step closer to freeing yourself from the cycle of your obsessions and compulsions. With one obsession out of the way, it's time to move on to the next one.

I am now able to prepare a meal for my family and friends in 30 to 60 minutes. I no longer worry that my cooking may cause harm to them and don't feel the urge to check the food repeatedly for signs of contamination.

My relationship with my family and friends has also improved over the past few weeks. I feel like I can enjoy the time I spend with them more than I did before.

Tracking Your Progress

Date	Exposure (Note if Imaginal or Real)	Discomfort (0 – 10) Beginning of Session	Feelings/Emotions	Physical Symptoms	Discomfort (0 – 10) End of Session

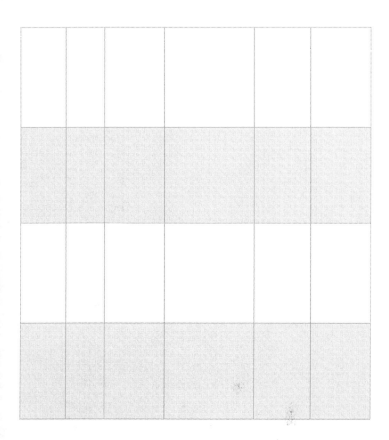

Challenging Your Faulty Beliefs

Once you have successfully gotten a handle on your anxiety, you are ready to move on to the next phase of treatment. Namely, we will be revisiting Cognitive Therapy, another old friend of ours from chapter 7.

As before, we will be using CT to help you identify cognitive distortions and other negative thought patterns. Once identified, these negative thought patterns are replaced with rational ways of thinking through cognitive restructuring. For example, in the context of hyper-responsibility, CT might be used to challenge the individual's role in the happiness and wellbeing of others.

Try as we may, we cannot always guarantee the welfare of those around us. After all, multiple factors contribute to a person's wellbeing, many of which are beyond our control. Therefore, learning to recognize the things that are beyond our control can be a critical step in reshaping your role in the responsibility of others.

Additionally, no one is perfect. We cannot always guarantee that we won't make a mistake or cause harm to someone else. To err is to be human, after all. Most of the time, we don't intend to cause harm to other people, and even when we do, it doesn't necessarily make us a bad person. Coming to terms with this can be a particularly difficult pill to swallow for those with hyper-responsibility.

Reshaping Your Role in the Responsibility of Others

Now it's time to explore your negative thought patterns in greater detail. To do so, we will be utilizing two powerful Cognitive Therapy techniques. The first is a Dysfunctional Thought Record. The second is another familiar face – Socratic Questioning.

Creating a Dysfunctional Thought Record

A Dysfunctional Thought Record is used to help you identify your negative thoughts and their causes. Once you have a better understanding of what provokes these thoughts, it becomes much easier to challenge and replace them with more rational ways of thinking.

Over the next few pages, you will find a Dysfunctional Thought Record worksheet to assist you in this endeavor.

Dysfunctional Thought Record Worksheet

Negative Thought	Cause	Emotions Experienced	Cognitive Distortion	Rational Thought	Outcome
Describe your thought in detail. On a scale of 1 – 10, how much did you believe it?	What triggered the thought? Describe the context.	What emotions did you experience? Rate the intensity of your emotions from 1 – 10.	What cognitive distortion does this thought represent?	Challenge the negative thought. Identify a rational thought to counter it.	Reevaluate how much you believe the negative thought (1 – 10) at the end of the exercise.

Socratic Questioning

Socratic Questioning is a particularly powerful technique when it comes to cognitive restructuring, which is why we are revisiting it in this chapter. Recall that Socratic Questioning is used to identify and challenge negative patterns of thought so that they may be replaced with more rational ways of thinking.

As before, we have included a Socratic Questioning worksheet for you to work through.

Socratic Questioning Worksheet

Thoughts are powerful things. They can shape the way we feel and even determine how we act. When thoughts become negative or harmful, it's important to challenge them and replace them with healthier thinking patterns.

Take a moment to answer each of the questions below. Try to spend at least 1 to 3 minutes considering each question (or longer if necessary) and be thoughtful in your responses.

Thought to be questioned:

Is there any evidence to support this thought? What is the evidence against it?

Are these thoughts based on facts or feelings?

Could I be misinterpreting something?

Am I making assumptions or jumping to conclusions?

Would other people interpret this situation differently? If so, how would they interpret it?

Am I considering all the evidence, or am I only looking at the evidence that supports my thought?

Does this thought represent a likely scenario, or am I catastrophizing?

Summing Up Hyper-responsibility

Overcoming hyper-responsibility isn't something that happens overnight. Any process that encourages you to change the way you think and behave will invariably be difficult. It will be uncomfortable (especially at first), and it will take time. With perseverance and hard work, however, it is possible to break free from this cycle.

Chapter 12: OCD-Related Hoarding

What is OCD-Related Hoarding?

For some, the obsessions and compulsions associated with OCD can cause difficulty in both the acquisition and discarding of items or possessions, irrespective of the item's actual value. Any attempt to part with the item causes significant distress. As a result, living areas may become cluttered, and in severe cases, may even pose potential health and safety hazards to those living in the structure. For example, large stacks of items may collapse on top of a person, pinning or crushing them beneath the rubble. Heavily cluttered areas may become fire hazards, and unsanitary living conditions can pose significant health risks to inhabitants.

It's important to note that hoarding OCD is considered a separate entity from Hoarding Disorder. While there are certain similarities between the two, there are also considerable differences, as we'll discuss below.

What's the Difference Between Hoarding Disorder and Hoarding OCD?

In the past, Hoarding Disorder (also known as Compulsive Hoarding,) was considered to be a subtype of OCD. As our understanding of both OCD and hoarding grew, however, it became clear that there were significant differences between the two disorders. The *Diagnostic and Statistical Manual of Mental Disorders, Fifth Edition* (DSM-5) now lists Hoarding Disorder as a separate entity from OCD-related hoarding. With that being said, it is possible to have both OCD and Hoarding Disorder. However, the diagnosis of either OCD or Hoarding Disorder is best left to a mental health professional such as a Psychiatrist, Psychologist, or therapist.

OCD-Related Hoarding

One important distinction is that the hoarding behaviors observed in OCD are driven by intrusive and distressing obsessions. To neutralize these uncomfortable thoughts and impulses, the individual engages in compulsive behaviors, such as the accumulation of large quantities of items that are typically of little to no value.

For example, a man with hoarding OCD might be overwhelmed by the feeling that something horrible will happen if he throws out his old magazines. Gradually, the magazines begin to stack up around his house until he can only navigate through small, cramped pathways between all of the clutter. His hoarding eventually gets so out of hand that his family stops visiting him altogether, and his relationship with them deteriorates.

Other manifestations of hoarding OCD include the following:

- A feeling of loss or incompleteness if a certain item were to be thrown away, such as a favorite childhood toy, may provoke hoarding behaviors.
- Fear of contamination may lead to the accumulation of large amounts of junk, garbage, or other items on the person's floor. In this case, the item becomes 'contaminated' once it makes contact with the ground. To prevent themselves from becoming similarly 'contaminated,' the individual avoids touching the item and leaves it on the ground.
- Contamination based obsessions may also be spurred by a need to protect other people from becoming contaminated. For example, when

shopping for food at a grocery store, a person might buy everything that they had touched. By touching an item, they believe that they have 'contaminated' it. To protect other people from becoming 'contaminated' therefore, they feel obligated to buy the object.

- A fear of discarding an item incorrectly or of potentially needing an item in the future can lead to the accumulation of useless items (magazines, newspapers, books, old food, clothing, cans, broken items, etc.)
- Belief in 'magical' or 'lucky numbers' may compel a person to buy large quantities of an item in multiples of their 'magical' or 'lucky number.'

Compared with Hoarding Disorder, people with OCD-related hoarding derive no pleasure from the act of hoarding. The resulting clutter may also become a significant source of distress and pose potential hazards to both health and safety. The individual's social, occupational, financial, and personal life can be impacted as well. Unsafe living conditions can place a strain on relationships and, in extreme cases, cause legal problems.

Additionally, those with hoarding OCD generally don't develop an attachment to the items or possessions they collect. They are also more likely to accumulate unusual items such as trash, used diapers, and rotten food.

Hoarding Disorder

In contrast, those with Hoarding Disorder do not suffer from intrusive, disturbing obsessions. Thoughts related to hoarding are not distressing and may even elicit feelings of excitement and pleasure. Moreover, hoarding behaviors are not undertaken to neutralize unwanted thoughts or impulses. Rather, the individual accumulates items as doing so brings them joy.

The items or possessions themselves are also deemed to have aesthetic value (although most people would deem them to be of limited or no value). This is an important distinction as those with hoarding OCD don't develop an attachment to the items they acquire. Therefore, any distress experienced when a person with hoarding OCD tries to discard an item is related to their obsessions rather than the loss of the item. On the other hand, a person with Hoarding Disorder experiences significant distress when parting with an item due to the emotional attachment they have for their possessions.

This is not to say that individuals with Hoarding Disorder don't experience any negative emotions as a result of their condition. Rather, it is the byproduct of their hoarding (clutter, social/financial/legal issues) which causes them distress.

Treatment Strategies

Cognitive Behavioral Therapy is the treatment of choice for both Hoarding Disorder and hoarding OCD. Depending on the condition being treated, the focus of CBT may differ. For example, when used to treat hoarding OCD, CBT is used to target the underlying obsessions and compulsions at the heart of the disorder.

Keep in mind that the successful treatment of hoarding OCD takes time. Typically the therapy is carried out over a period of months under the supervision of a specialized mental health clinician. Sessions are held both at the clinician's office and the individual's house. Given the nature of OCD-related hoarding, the treatment should ideally be carried out under the supervision of a mental health clinician. Depending on your location and access to mental health providers, however, this may not be feasible. In these circumstances, CBT may be used by other health professionals, novice therapists, or laypersons with an understanding of OCD-related hoarding and the therapy methods used to treat it.

Before you create your treatment plan, however, it may be helpful to gauge the impact hoarding has had on your life. Take a few minutes to fill out the Hoarding Impact Worksheet below. We also recommend filling out the worksheet approximately halfway through the treatment process and again at the end. This will allow you to monitor your progress and can be used as a motivational tool as you work your way through the program.

Once you have filled out the Hoarding Impact Worksheet, you're ready to develop your treatment plan. We'll start by utilizing ERP to tackle the obsessions and compulsions unique to hoarding OCD. Initially, our goal will be to prevent the acquisition of new items. Afterward, we will gradually work our way through the process of decluttering.

To wrap things up, we'll take another look at CT to address any cognitive distortions or negative thought patterns that may be fueling your hoarding behaviors.

Hoarding Impact Worksheet

1. Do you currently have a problem with collecting or buying more things than you need? If so, has this had an impact on you financially?

2. Are you experiencing difficulty discarding items that most people would normally get rid of? If so, what items do you tend to hold onto? Why do you feel compelled to keep those items?

3. How has the clutter impacted your ability to use the rooms in your home/apartment?

4. Describe the impact your hoarding behaviors, and clutter have had on you emotionally.

5. Have the hoarding behaviors and clutter impaired your ability to live your day-to-day life? Consider the impact this has had on your social/family life, finances, daily routine, and work/school.

6. Imagine your house/apartment free of clutter. Describe what it would look like. What would it mean to you for your home to be free from clutter?

Exposure and Response Prevention Revisited

By now, you're likely well-acquainted with Exposure and Response Prevention Therapy. If not (or if you would like a quick refresher,) head over to chapter 5 for a bit of background on this powerful treatment modality.

The treatment process for hoarding OCD can be a particularly stressful one, which is why we have broken it down into separate phases. In a process similar to the treatment for Hoarding Disorder, we will start by showing you how to overcome the urge to acquire new items. Then we will guide you through the process of decluttering your home.

Prevention of Acquisition

As before, we have included an ERP worksheet below so that you may develop your personalized treatment plan. A sample plan has also been included for your review. Before starting, consider all of the ways you acquire new items (in the context of hoarding). It may be helpful to write them down in the order you plan on tackling them. We recommend starting with the method of acquisition that you think will be the least distressing to address and working your way up from there.

Your ERP plan will ultimately be determined by the way(s) in which you acquire new items. For example, if you experience the impulse to buy an article of clothing after touching it, your ERP session might consist of you touching a piece of merchandise without purchasing it. Similarly, if your OCD-related hoarding centers around fears of contamination, your ERP session might involve holding the contaminated object in your hand without engaging in your normal compulsive responses, such as avoiding contact with the item or handwashing.

Remember that your ERP sessions should last anywhere from 60 to 90 minutes. To ensure that your sessions are effective, expect to continue the exposure until you experience at least a 50% reduction in your anxiety.

ERP for Acquisition Prevention

The following worksheet can be used as a guide to create a personalized ERP plan. At the end of the worksheet, you will find a chart to document your progress over time. Remember that this is a gradual process, so don't get discouraged if you don't notice an improvement in your symptoms right away!

Step 1: Setting Realistic Goals

Make a list of your obsessions. Start with the obsession that is the least distressing and work your way up to the most uncomfortable. Ranking each obsession using a 0 – 10 numeric scale may be helpful. Take note of your list, as this is the order you will be completing them in.

Step 2: Imaginal Exposure/Exposure Therapy

Visualize the trigger in your mind to start. Writing the content of your obsession down or making an audio recording of yourself may also be helpful. When you feel you are ready, move on to confronting the trigger in real life. Pay close attention to what you are feeling, both emotionally and physically.

What feelings are you experiencing?

Are you experiencing any physical symptoms?

Step 3: Response Prevention

Refrain from giving in to your compulsive thoughts and behaviors. Don't try to distract yourself or avoid facing the trigger. Acknowledge both the trigger and the feelings and sensations that come with it. Remember, the short term discomfort is well worth the long term gain of being freed from the cycle of your obsessions and compulsions! Don't seek reassurance either, as reassurance interferes with the recovery process. Continue the session until you experience at least a 50% reduction in your symptoms.

Step 4: Keep With It!

Try to be consistent with your sessions. Remember that sessions may take 60 minutes or longer, especially when first starting. Over time, you should notice a gradual decrease in your symptoms. By the end of treatment, the same triggers that were so distressing before should evoke little to no response.

Step 5: You Did It!

Congratulations, you made it! All that hard work has finally paid off, and you are one step closer to freeing yourself from the cycle of your obsessions and compulsions. With one obsession out of the way, it's time to move on to the next one.

ERP for Acquisition Prevention (Sample)

Name Stephan V.

Step 1: Setting Realistic Goals

Make a list of your obsessions. Start with the obsession that is the least distressing and work your way up to the most uncomfortable. Ranking each obsession using a 0 – 10 numeric scale may be helpful. Take note of your list, as this is the order you will be completing them in.

Whenever I go shopping for clothes, I get the distressing urge to buy every article of clothing that I touch, regardless of whether I want the item or not. I'm so afraid that if I don't, someone else will come into contact with the item and become "contaminated." As a result, my apartment has become overrun by clothes that I don't want and don't use. My spending has also put my finances in a precarious position. I'm behind on my rent and don't have the money I need to pay my bills.

My level of discomfort is 9/10.

Step 2: Imaginal Exposure/Exposure Therapy

Visualize the trigger in your mind to start. Writing the content of your obsession down or making an audio recording of yourself may also be helpful. When you feel you are ready, move on to confronting the trigger in real life. Pay close attention to what you are feeling, both emotionally and physically.

Imaginal Exposure*: I visualize myself in my local mall. From the entrance, I make my way into one of the clothing stores and begin to browse around. Normally, I would try to avoid touching things, but this time, I force myself to pick up a pair of jeans. I hold the object in my hands briefly before returning it to its original place.*

I glance at the object one more time before forcing myself to walk away. I'm feeling anxious. My mind is telling me to go back and purchase the item, but I know that I can't give in to my obsessions if I want to overcome my OCD. As uncomfortable as it feels, I allow myself to experience these thoughts and emotions without acting on them.

What feelings are you experiencing?

I feel extremely anxious. I'm so worried that I may "contaminate" someone else who comes into contact with the pair of jeans that I touched. What if someone gets seriously ill because I didn't buy that pair of jeans?

Are you experiencing any physical symptoms?

I can feel my heart racing in my chest. The anxiety is so intense that I almost feel nauseous.

Exposure Therapy: *Once I have gotten a better handle on my anxiety through imaginal exposure, I will visit a clothing store in real life. While I am in the store, I will physically handle an article of clothing without giving in to my compulsion to buy it afterward.*

Step 3: Response Prevention

Refrain from giving in to your compulsive thoughts and behaviors. Don't try to distract yourself or avoid facing the trigger. Acknowledge both the trigger and the feelings and sensations that come with it. Remember, the short term discomfort is well worth the long term gain of being freed from the cycle of your obsessions and compulsions! Don't seek reassurance either, as reassurance interferes with the recovery process. Continue the session until you experience at least a 50% reduction in your symptoms.

While I am in the clothing store, I will place all articles of clothing that I touch back on their shelves/displays. Most importantly, I will NOT buy any items that I touch.

Step 4: Keep With It!

Try to be consistent with your sessions. Remember that sessions may take 60 minutes or longer, especially when first starting. Over time, you should notice a gradual decrease in your symptoms. By the end of treatment, the same triggers that were so distressing before should evoke little to no response.

I have noticed a slight decline in my symptoms over the past few weeks. Initially, I was experiencing 9/10 discomfort when shopping for clothes. Now, I am experiencing 4/10 discomfort.

Step 5: You Did It!

Congratulations, you made it! All that hard work has finally paid off, and you are one step closer to freeing yourself from the cycle of your obsessions and compulsions. With one obsession out of the way, it's time to move on to the next one.

I can hardly believe it, but I made it! I will admit, it was hard and very, very uncomfortable at first, but it was worth it in the end. I can now go shopping for clothes and handle items without buying them. Most of the time, I don't experience any distressing thoughts or urges.

Even when I do, they are usually so minuscule that I hardly notice them.

Tracking Your Progress

Date	Exposure (Note if Imaginal or Real)	Discomfort (0 – 10) Beginning of Session	Feelings/Emotions	Physical Symptoms	Discomfort (0 – 10) End of Session

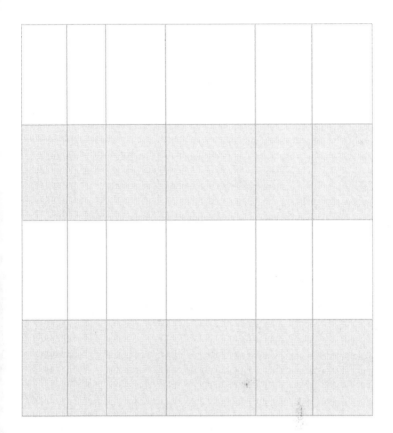

The Process of Decluttering

Before starting the process of sorting and decluttering, it may be helpful to formulate a "plan of attack," so to speak. For example, what will you do with the items you discard? Do you plan on donating them? If so, where do you plan to take the items? If the items aren't suitable to donate, how will you dispose of them (i.e., trash or recycling)? To keep yourself on track it may be helpful to focus your efforts on one room at a time. Start with smaller ERP sessions and work your way up to bigger challenges (such as decluttering entire rooms). Only handle each item once, sort it, and move on to the next one.

Having the support and assistance of family and friends during this time can be helpful. You may even choose to create a decluttering team of trusted individuals to assist you. To keep things running smoothly, make sure that everyone is on the same page. When the time comes to start sorting and discarding items, however, you are the one who must make the decisions. Your decluttering team may assist you in this process but is not allowed to make decisions regarding the items in your house.

As before, this process will be guided by your obsessions and compulsions. For example, if you get the feeling that something terrible will happen should you get rid of an item, then your ERP session would consist of you discarding it. Afterward, you would allow yourself to acknowledge and experience the resulting anxiety until you experienced at least a 50% reduction of your anxiety.

On the following pages, you will find a sample ERP plan to help guide you in this process. Should you require a blank copy of the worksheet, please refer to the one provided earlier in the chapter.

ERP for Decluttering (Sample)

Name Michael A.

Step 1: Setting Realistic Goals

Make a list of your obsessions. Start with the obsession that is the least distressing and work your way up to the most uncomfortable. Ranking each obsession using a 0 – 10 numeric scale may be helpful. Take note of your list, as this is the order you will be completing them in.

Whenever I try to throw out a newspaper, magazine, or book, I am overwhelmed by the feeling that something horrible will happen if I get rid of the item. As a result, it has been easier (in terms of my anxiety) to keep these items rather than throw them away. It's gotten to the point where I can barely move around my house.

My level of discomfort is 8/10.

Step 2: Imaginal Exposure/Exposure Therapy

Visualize the trigger in your mind to start. Writing the content of your obsession down or making an audio recording of yourself may also be helpful. When you feel you are ready, move on to confronting the trigger in real life. Pay close attention to what you are feeling, both emotionally and physically.

Exposure Therapy*: Depending on the condition of a book or magazine, I will either donate it or throw it out. I will also throw out all newspapers.*

To start, I have selected a small stack of 2-3 books. Depending on the book's condition, I will place it in the donation pile or discard pile.

What feelings are you experiencing?

I feel terrified. I'm not sure what will happen after getting rid of the books. I'm really worried that something awful is going to happen.

Are you experiencing any physical symptoms?

I feel jittery, like I can't sit still.

Step 3: Response Prevention

Refrain from giving in to your compulsive thoughts and behaviors. Don't try to distract yourself or avoid facing the trigger. Acknowledge both the trigger and the feelings and sensations that come with it. Remember, the short term discomfort is well worth the long term gain of being freed from the cycle of your obsessions and compulsions! Don't seek reassurance either, as reassurance interferes with the recovery process. Continue the session until you experience at least a 50% reduction in your symptoms.

I will leave the books in the donation/discard piles and will get rid of them as appropriate.

Step 4: Keep With It!

Try to be consistent with your sessions. Remember that sessions may take 60 minutes or longer, especially when first starting. Over time, you should notice a gradual decrease in your symptoms. By the end of treatment, the same triggers that were so distressing before should evoke little to no response.

Over the past few weeks, my hoarding symptoms have gotten better. Initially, I was experiencing 8/10 discomfort when getting rid of items. Now, my level of discomfort has decreased to 3/10.

I feel like I am ready to challenge myself a little bit more. During my next session, I will aim to declutter my living room.

Step 5: You Did It!

Congratulations, you made it! All that hard work has finally paid off, and you are one step closer to freeing yourself from the cycle of your obsessions and compulsions. With one obsession out of the way, it's time to move on to the next one.

It took time, but I have successfully decluttered my entire house. For the first time in years, I can move freely from room to room and perform my everyday activities without difficulty.
I am no longer afraid to have friends and family over and have even held dinner parties at my house.

Cognitive Therapy for Hoarding OCD

As we discussed previously, our thoughts have a profound impact on our feelings and emotions. If we frequently engage in negative self-talk, we are more likely to experience negative emotions such as anxiety, stress, anger, or sadness. We may even start to think of ourselves in a harsh, overly critical way.

If these thoughts become powerful enough, we may even start to believe that they are true, regardless of whether they are or not. These thoughts and emotions can then become a key driver of anxiety disorders such as OCD, Generalized Anxiety, and Social Anxiety. This is true of OCD-related hoarding as well. In this case, the underlying obsessions lead to compulsive hoarding behaviors.

Cognitive Restructuring

Recall that cognitive restructuring teaches us to challenge our negative thought patterns and replace them with more realistic ways of thinking. In the context of anxiety disorders (such as OCD), cognitive restructuring may be used to help us disengage from our anxiety and replace irrational thoughts with more realistic ones.

By emphasizing observation, cognitive restructuring also encourages us to be more compassionate and empathetic, especially to ourselves.

To this end, we will be returning to a helpful tool of ours from chapter 7: The Thought Journal. You should use this exercise whenever a negative thought or feeling is identified. Admittedly, this can be a challenge, especially when first starting. For some individuals, their negative thought patterns are so ingrained in the way they think they may not even realize they are falling into the trap of cognitive distortions.

Changing the way you think will take time and practice, but it is possible. Remember to be patient with yourself. Don't get discouraged if you don't notice any results right away. During the first couple of weeks, we recommend using the Thought Journal provided for your exercises. As you progress, you should be able to move through the exercise entirely in your mind.

To start the exercise, consider the event that triggered the automatic thought. What feelings or emotions were you experiencing? What was your response? Lastly, counter your automatic thought with a rational thought. Once you have completed the exercise, it may be helpful to reevaluate your emotions. Most of the time, you should notice at least a moderate reduction in the intensity of your emotions.

Event	Thought	Feeling	Behavior	Rational Counterstatement
Example: I accidentally touched a jacket in a store that I know I can't afford.	I have contaminated the jacket. If I don't buy it, I could be responsible for contaminating someone else and making them sick.	I'm very worried that I might make someone else ill. I can feel my anxiety building the more I	I placed the jacket in my cart even though I know I can't afford it.	I practice very good hand hygiene, so it is highly unlikely that I have contaminated the jacket. Moreover, it's improbable that someone will get ill after touching the item.

think
about
it.

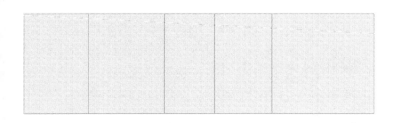

Wrapping Things Up

OCD-related hoarding can be a challenging condition to treat. With time, patience, and the proper treatment, however, it is possible to take back control of your life (and your house).

Given the complex nature of hoarding OCD, we have included the name of an organization that may prove beneficial as you move through the self-directed treatment program outlined in this chapter. This resource will also be provided in chapter 16, Getting Help.

Resources for OCD-Related Hoarding

The International OCD Foundation has a resource directory that can be used to find therapists, treatment programs, and clinics that specialize in hoarding in your area. They also offer webinars on the disorder (as well as other disorders related to OCD). More information can be found on their website: Home - Hoarding (iocdf.org).

Chapter 13: Hypochondriasis

What is Health Anxiety?

Health anxiety, also known as hypochondriasis, is a disorder characterized by the obsessive belief that one has or that one may develop a serious illness. For some individuals, this preoccupation (in addition to the anxiety that comes with it) can be crippling. In many cases, it may impair a person's ability to function in school, work, or social settings.

In this chapter, we will explore hypochondriasis and its relationship with OCD. To round things off, we'll delve into the treatment strategies that are currently available for this condition.

The Role of Anxiety in Hypochondriasis

While it may not seem like it at times, anxiety is not necessarily a bad thing. For example, consider the following hypothetical scenario: Imagine yourself taking a leisurely stroll through a forest. For the moment, you feel completely at ease with your surroundings. That is until you spot a large black bear lumbering down the hiking trail towards you. Upon seeing the large predator, your body activates its "fight or flight" response. Almost immediately, you feel your muscles tense. Your breath quickens, and you can feel your heart racing in your chest as your body prepares you for whatever happens next.

Undoubtedly, the anxiety and fear experienced in this scenario are far from pleasant. However, these emotions and the physical responses that come with them play a vital role in our ability to identify and respond to potential sources of danger. When our "anxiety response" becomes overactive, as it does with hypochondriasis, it can have a detrimental effect on our physical and mental wellbeing.

In hypochondriasis, people develop a hyperawareness of their bodily sensations and physical symptoms. Normal body sensations such as changes in heart rate, breathing, visual acuity, and balance may be misinterpreted as signs of a terrible disease. In this case, their "anxiety response" becomes falsely activated by a perceived threat, when, in reality, there is no real danger.

Other fears commonly observed in health anxiety include the following:

- Fear of dying from a serious illness or disease.

- Fear of prolonged or permanent mental or physical suffering.
- Fear that you won't receive the correct diagnosis or treatment for your symptoms
- Fear that you will leave your loved ones behind because you failed to take care of yourself.

So, we know what hypochondriasis is, but what causes people with the disorder to misinterpret their physical symptoms when, in reality, there is most likely no cause for concern? Admittedly, part of the problem may lie with a person's inherent beliefs about health and wellness. For example, people with health anxiety may hold very strict beliefs of what they consider to be "good health." Any deviation from this is then misinterpreted as a sign of "bad health." In other cases, a person's beliefs may be driven by negative or traumatic past experiences. For example, consider the case of an individual who lost a parent to cancer. Following the loss of their loved one, they might start to believe that it is only a matter of time before they are diagnosed with cancer as well.

Compulsive Responses and Reassurance Seeking Behaviors

In an attempt to alleviate their anxiety, individuals with hypochondriasis often engage in reassurance-seeking behaviors. For example, to reassure themselves that they are not seriously ill, a person may repeatedly call their physician, schedule appointments, or routinely visit their local emergency room.

Given the wealth of information available online and the relative ease of accessing it, it's not uncommon for those with hypochondriasis to spend hours googling or researching various symptoms and diseases. Unfortunately, more information is not always a good thing. Rather than providing reassurance, this behavior only reinforces unhealthy ways of thinking and perpetuates the cycle of anxiety-provoking thoughts, followed by compulsive reassurance seeking.

Other reassurance-seeking behaviors and compulsive behaviors observed in health anxiety include:

- Performing frequent body checks or examinations.
- Frequently monitoring vital signs such as heart rate and blood pressure.

- Asking family or friends to examine you.
- Seeking the advice of family or friends.
- Actively avoiding objects or places where you may be exposed to germs or illnesses.
- Repeatedly reviewing behaviors to make sure the appropriate precautions were taken.

While reassurance-seeking behaviors may allay their anxiety, the relief provided is temporary. Ultimately, the fear of serious illness resurfaces, prompting the individual to seek reassurance once more. This creates a vicious cycle of anxiety and reassurance seeking that can significantly impair a person's ability to function and place strain on relationships.

Health Anxiety and OCD – What's the Difference?

There's no denying that hypochondriasis and OCD share certain similarities. As we know, OCD is characterized by obsessions and compulsions. In some respects, the near-constant fear of having some terrible illness is akin to the obsessive thoughts seen in OCD. Attempts to seek reassurance from medical professionals, loved ones, or other resources (books, journals, websites, etc.) are similar to checking compulsions in OCD. In both cases,

the compulsions or attempts to seek reassurance also fail
to relieve the individual's anxiety.

Despite these similarities, OCD and hypochondriasis are
considered separate disorders. However, there is some
debate about whether health anxiety should be
considered a subtype of OCD.

Regardless, there are also important differences between
the two disorders. For example, individuals with health
anxiety exhibit more fear of their bodily sensations and
physical symptoms. Moreover, they may be less aware of
the fact that their fears are irrational and have less
insight into their condition compared to those with OCD.
This is not to say that hypochondriasis and OCD are
mutually exclusive of one another, as an individual with
OCD may also be diagnosed with health anxiety and vise
versa.

Treatment Options

As with OCD, the mainstay of treatment for health
anxiety is CBT. The goal of therapy, in this case, is to help
modify a person's misinterpretations of harmless bodily
sensations and eliminate reassurance seeking and

compulsive behaviors. Generally, this is achieved using a combination of ERP and Cognitive Therapy.

ERP for Health Anxiety

During Exposure and Response Prevention Therapy you will be tasked with confronting the scenarios and bodily sensations that you would normally attempt to avoid. The intention is to provoke the anxiety or fear response that typically accompanies the exposure.

Over time (and with a little help from our good friend habituation,) you will learn to acknowledge your physical sensations without fear or the need to dwell on them. At the same time, you will learn to accept the uncertainty about the meaning of your physical sensations (i.e., do they truly represent a symptom or not). Your ERP plan will naturally depend on your fears and compulsive responses. When drafting your plan, you may consider the following examples or simply create your own plan, depending on your needs.

Examples of ERP Plans for Health Anxiety:
- For fears centered around contamination, exposure might consist of exposing oneself to the feared setting, object, situation, etc.

- Writing an imaginal story where you have a serious or terminal illness and the consequences that would arise from this.
- Writing an imaginal story where you fail to take the necessary precautions to prevent an illness.
- Watch a video or movie about a person with a serious or terminal illness.
- Read articles or stories about a person with a serious or terminal illness.

This list is far from exhaustive, but it may be a helpful reference as you draft your ERP plan. On the following pages, you will find the familiar ERP worksheet along with a sample plan. Once you have successfully created your ERP plan, you will be ready to move on to the next step.

ERP for Health Anxiety

The following worksheet can be used as a guide to create a personalized ERP plan. At the end of the worksheet, you will find a chart to document your progress over time. Remember that this is a gradual process, so don't get discouraged if you don't notice an improvement in your symptoms right away!

Step 1: Setting Realistic Goals

Consider your fears regarding your physical symptoms and what they might mean. Start with the fear that is the least distressing and work your way up to the most uncomfortable. Ranking each fear using a 0 – 10 numeric scale may be helpful. Take note of your list, as this is the order you will be completing them in.

Step 2: Imaginal Exposure/Exposure Therapy

Visualize the trigger in your mind to start. Writing the content of your fear down or making an audio recording of yourself may also be helpful. When you feel you are ready, move on to confronting the trigger in real life. Pay close attention to what you are feeling, both emotionally and physically.

What feelings are you experiencing?

Are you experiencing any physical symptoms?

Step 3: Response Prevention

Refrain from giving in to your compulsive behaviors. Don't try to distract yourself or avoid facing the trigger. Acknowledge both the trigger and the feelings and sensations that come with it. Remember, the short term discomfort is well worth the long term gain of being freed from the cycle of your anxiety and compulsive behaviors! Don't seek reassurance either, as reassurance interferes with the recovery process. Continue the session until you experience at least a 50% reduction in your symptoms.

Step 4: Keep With It!

Try to be consistent with your sessions. Remember that sessions may take 60 minutes or longer, especially when first starting. Over time, you should notice a gradual decrease in your symptoms. By the end of treatment, the same triggers that were so distressing before should evoke little to no response.

Step 5: You Did It!

Congratulations, you made it! All that hard work has finally paid off, and you are one step closer to freeing yourself from the cycle of your fears and compulsive responses.

ERP for Health Anxiety (Sample)

Name Zachary S.

Step 1: Setting Realistic Goals

Consider your fears regarding your physical symptoms and what they might mean. Start with the fear that is the least distressing and work your way up to the most uncomfortable. Ranking each fear using a 0 – 10 numeric scale may be helpful. Take note of your list, as this is the order you will be completing them in.

Sometimes I get this sharp pain in my left arm. It doesn't last long, but I'm afraid it might be a sign of something serious. I've heard that some people get referred pain in their left arm when they have a heart attack. Could my arm pain be a sign of a heart attack?

My level of discomfort is 10/10.

Step 2: Imaginal Exposure/Exposure Therapy

Visualize the trigger in your mind to start. Writing the content of your fear down or making an audio recording of yourself may also be helpful. When you feel you are ready, move on to confronting the trigger in real life. Pay close attention to what you are feeling, both emotionally and physically.

Imaginal Exposure/Exposure Therapy: During my ERP session, I will create an imaginal story in which I am diagnosed with a heart attack. I will consider the consequences of this diagnosis and what it might mean for my future.

What feelings are you experiencing?

I feel very anxious.

Are you experiencing any physical symptoms?

My heart is racing so fast I'm afraid it might burst from my chest. The palms of my hands feel sweaty, and I'm struck with a sense of nausea.

Step 3: Response Prevention

Refrain from giving in to your compulsive behaviors. Don't try to distract yourself or avoid facing the trigger. Acknowledge both the trigger and the feelings and sensations that come with it. Remember, the short term discomfort is well worth the long term gain of being freed from the cycle of your anxiety and compulsive behaviors! Don't seek reassurance either, as reassurance interferes with the recovery process. Continue the session until you experience at least a 50% reduction in your symptoms.

I will refrain from researching my symptoms on Google. Additionally, I won't seek reassurance from my doctor or significant other.

Step 4: Keep With It!

Try to be consistent with your sessions. Remember that sessions may take 60 minutes or longer, especially when first starting. Over time, you should notice a gradual decrease in your symptoms. By the end of treatment, the same triggers that were so distressing before should evoke little to no response.

I have noticed a steady decrease in my symptoms over the past month or so. Now, when I create my imaginal story, I don't get as anxious. Additionally, when I experience arm pain in real life, I can resist the urge to research my symptoms or seek reassurance most of the time.

Step 5: You Did It!

Congratulations, you made it! All that hard work has finally paid off, and you are one step closer to freeing yourself from the cycle of your fears and compulsive responses.

I made it to the end of my ERP treatment plan. It was difficult at first, but I am so glad I followed it through to the end. Now, when I experience the arm pain, I can accept the pain for what it is, along with the uncertainty that comes with it. I no longer feel afraid of this pain and don't feel the need to research my symptoms or seek reassurance from others.

Tracking Your Progress

Date	Exposure (Note if Imaginal or Real)	Discomfort (0 – 10) Beginning of Session	Feelings/Emotions	Physical Symptoms	Discomfort (0 – 10) End of Session

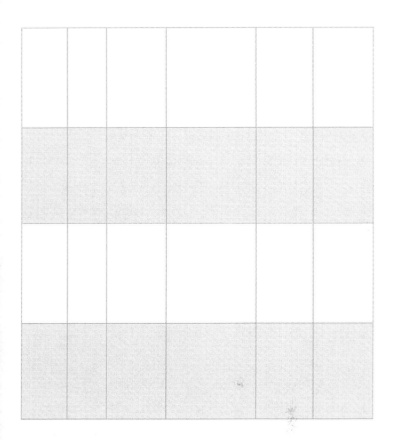

Guided Discovery Through Cognitive Therapy

Now that you have created your ERP plan, it's time to modify how you perceive and interpret your physical sensations. To accomplish this goal, we will engage in the process of cognitive restructuring once more. In particular, we will utilize cognitive restructuring to address four of the most commonly encountered inaccurate beliefs that act as the driving force behind health anxiety.

You are completely responsible for taking all necessary steps to prevent illness: While it is important to practice good health habits such as eating a varied diet rich in fruits and veggies, getting 7-9 hours of sleep per night, etc., there is a point where illness prevention can become unnecessarily excessive. Realistically, if you took every precaution possible to prevent illness, it's unlikely you would ever be able to leave your house. The truth is, most things in life (even the enjoyable things) come with some level of risk.

Your symptoms and physical sensations are indicative of an illness or disease and always have an identifiable cause: Our bodies constantly produce various physical sensations whether we are aware of them or not. Occasionally, these symptoms may be indicative of a health concern; however, most of the time, they aren't indicative of anything. Learning to accept this uncertainty can be particularly challenging; however, it is a pivotal step in the recovery process.

It is possible to know the status of your health with complete certainty: Unfortunately, this is simply not possible. Uncertainty is a fact of life, after all, as much as we might wish otherwise. While it's not possible to have 100% control over your health, you do have the power to choose how to live your life. Accepting this is an important step in taking back your life.

Receiving the correct diagnosis will always lead to the appropriate treatment and complete resolution of your symptoms: Despite recent advances in the medical field, we don't have a definitive cure or treatment for all symptoms or diseases. For example, consider a chronic medical condition such as Fibromyalgia, for which there is no universally accepted treatment.

Now that we have reviewed some of the most commonly encountered inaccurate beliefs in health anxiety, it's time for you to identify your negative thought patterns. Once again, we will be using the concept of Thought Journal. You should use this exercise whenever a negative thought, feeling, or physical sensation is identified.

During the first couple of weeks, we recommend using the Thought Journal provided for your exercises. As you progress, you should be able to move through the exercise entirely in your mind.

To start the exercise, consider the event or physical sensation that triggered the negative thought. What feelings or emotions were you experiencing? What was your response? Lastly, counter your negative thought with rational thought. Once you have completed the exercise, it may be helpful to reevaluate your emotions. Most of the time, you should notice at least a moderate reduction in the intensity of your emotions.

Event	Thought	Feeling	Behavior	Rational Counterstatement
Example: I've had a dry cough on and off since lunch today.	What if my cough is the result of a serious illness such as pneumonia or lung cancer?	I'm so anxious I can barely focus on anything else at work.	I repeatedly googled my symptoms when I should have been working.	The chances of my cough being the result of either illness are extremely low. Moreover, I don't have any other symptoms or risk factors.

Summing Things Up

Health anxiety can be a difficult mountain to climb. However, the fact that you have made it this far means that you are up to the challenge. In addition to the exercises provided in this self-help guide, you may wish to seek out the guidance of an experienced therapist. Group therapy, in particular, has shown promise in the treatment of health anxiety.

To this end, we recommend visiting the National Alliance on Mental Illness (NAMI) website. The organization offers a helpline that you can use to explore resources available in your area. Additionally, NAMI offers support groups for individuals with mental health conditions and their families. To find out more about NAMI, please refer to chapter 16, How to Get Help.

NAMI HelpLine: 1-800-950-NAMI (6264)

NAMI Support Groups: Support Groups | NAMI: National Alliance on Mental Illness

Chapter 14: Associated Conditions

It's not uncommon for a person with OCD to have at least one other mental health condition. In fact, a large-scale community study of mental health in U.S. adults showed that 90% of individuals with OCD reported having at least one other mental health condition.

Some of the most commonly encountered comorbid conditions include depression and anxiety disorders such as Generalized Anxiety Disorder, Social Anxiety, and Panic Disorder.

Depression

Odds are at one point in your life, you've gone through a rough patch or felt a little down. For those with Major Depressive Disorder, however, the feeling of hopelessness and despair goes well beyond this. It pervades every aspect of their lives and impacts their ability to function and carry out their day-to-day activities. Depression can also manifest in different ways, and symptoms may vary from one person to another.

Other symptoms of depression include:

- Changes in sleeping patterns (difficulty falling/staying asleep or sleeping too much.)
- Changes in appetite (eating too much or too little.)
- Difficulty concentrating.
- Fatigue or lack of energy.
- Loss of interest in activities the individual would normally enjoy.
- Feelings of hopelessness or guilt.
- Changes in movement (being so agitated that you are unable to sit still or being less active than usual.)
- Suicidal thoughts.

To meet the diagnostic criteria for major depression, the above symptoms must be present for at least two weeks and can last anywhere from a few months to years. Keep in mind, however, that only a licensed mental health professional can make the diagnosis of Major Depressive Disorder. If you are concerned that you may have depression, don't be afraid to reach out for help! Major depression is a serious mental health condition, but with the proper treatment, many people do get better and go on to lead fulfilling lives.

The Link Between Depression and OCD

It's estimated that around 60% of people with OCD will experience at least one episode of major depression in their lives. While the two conditions can "feed" off each other, the depression is usually secondary to the person's OCD. In other words, the individual's depression is a direct result of their OCD symptoms.

Anxiety Disorders

Anxiety is a normal part of our everyday lives. For example, think of a time, you had to get up and speak in front of a large group of people. While unpleasant, the anxiety triggered by this situation was not necessarily a bad thing (even if it didn't seem like it at the time.) It may have even motivated you to practice beforehand so that you could give your best performance. When our anxiety becomes persistent, overwhelming, and begins to impact our ability to perform our everyday activities, however, an anxiety disorder may be the culprit.

According to the National Alliance on Mental Illness (NAMI), "anxiety disorders are a group of related conditions, each having unique symptoms." All of the disorders are characterized by "persistent, excessive fear or worry in situations that are not threatening."

Symptoms commonly encountered in anxiety disorders include:

- Feelings of dread or apprehension.
- Feeling tense.
- Feelings of restlessness.
- Becoming easily irritated or angry.
- Anticipating the worst possible outcome.
- Being hypervigilant for signs of danger.
- Rapid heartbeat and shortness of breath.
- Sweating.
- Tremors or twitching.
- Fatigue or lack of energy.
- Difficulty falling or staying asleep.
- Headaches, upset stomach, diarrhea.

Types of Anxiety Disorders

While there are many types of anxiety disorders, we will only be covering a select few. In particular, we will briefly review three of the most commonly encountered conditions that overlap with OCD: Generalized Anxiety Disorder, Social Anxiety, and Panic Disorder.

Generalized Anxiety Disorder: GAD is characterized by persistent, excessive worrying about everyday life.

Often, the worry is present even in situations that would be considered non-threatening by most people. The individual may spend hours worrying and agonizing over various things throughout the day, making it difficult to function or perform their everyday tasks.

Social Anxiety Disorder: SAD is characterized by an intense fear of social interaction. In many cases, this disorder is driven by an irrational fear centered around humiliation (e.g., inadvertently offending someone or saying something stupid.) To avoid social interactions, the individual may refrain from participating in conversations or may self-isolate.

Panic Disorder: Panic Disorder is characterized by panic attacks that are accompanied by feelings of extreme terror or impending doom. Symptoms of a panic attack include chest pain, dizziness, palpitations, and shortness of breath. Often, the symptoms are significant enough that the individual may mistake them for a heart attack and seek emergency medical care. Additionally, the attacks can strike repeatedly and without warning. To avoid an attack, a person with Panic Disorder may take extreme measures such as social isolation.

If you are concerned that you may have an anxiety disorder, we strongly encourage you to reach out for help. Only a licensed mental health professional can diagnose you with an anxiety disorder. Additionally, a Psychiatrist or therapist may be able to offer additional treatments or resources not covered in this self-help guide. For information on how to find a mental health professional, please see chapter 16 of this book.

How to Approach Your Anxiety

We have covered a multitude of treatment strategies so far in this book, many of which can be successfully applied to the treatment of anxiety. To avoid being overly repetitious, we won't be reviewing those strategies here. However, we strongly encourage you to apply the therapies and techniques you have learned so far in the treatment of your anxiety.

To add another tool to your arsenal, we will briefly review Dialectical Behavioral Therapy (DBT) and its role in the treatment of anxiety.

Dialectical Behavioral Therapy

DBT is typically used in the treatment of Borderline Personality Disorder; however, it also has useful applications in the treatment of anxiety as well. Dialectical Behavioral Therapy is a type of CBT that utilizes mindfulness and meditation to help regulate our emotions and behaviors. By using these techniques, DBT helps us focus our mind on the present moment rather than the past or future. It also encourages us to relinquish our need for control and to accept and not dwell on the things that are out of our control, such as past events or another person's actions.

The following are three simple and quick DBT exercises that can be incorporated into your daily routine.

Mindfulness Eating: Pick a food that you enjoy and observe it closely. What does it feel like in your hands? Take note of its color, shape, and texture. Now turn your attention to its smell. Lastly, put a small piece of the food into your mouth. What does it taste like? What texture does it have?

Observe an Object: Find an object and pick it up in your hand. Focus all of your attention on it. What does the object look like? Take note of its shape, color, texture, and weight. While you do this, don't assess the object in any way. Simply observe it in your hand.

Observe Your Thoughts: Find a quiet and comfortable location where you won't be disturbed. Sit or lie down in a comfortable position and slowly release all of the tension in your body. Once you have done this, close your eyes and focus your attention on your breathing. Take note of how your body feels as you breathe in and out. Next, focus your attention on your thoughts. As each thought comes into your mind, acknowledge it for what it is, without judgment. Allow your thoughts to come and go in this manner, without dwelling on them. If you have difficulty with this, try picturing your thoughts as leaves floating down a stream or clouds passing through the sky.

If you become distracted or start to dwell on a thought, gently bring yourself back to the present moment. Continue to observe your thoughts for a few minutes. Once you feel you are ready, return your attention to your breathing before opening your eyes.

The above exercises are designed to help ground you in the present moment and can be used whenever you have a spare moment or are feeling anxious. As every individual is different, we encourage you to experiment with the DBT exercises provided (along with the other

CBT modalities discussed in this book) to find the exercises that work best for you.

Chapter 15: Living Your Best Life

Applying Your New Skills in Everyday Life

Taking the first step is often the hardest part. By making it this far, you have demonstrated your commitment to breaking free from your obsessions and compulsions and have taken that initial, critical step (and then some!) After completing this self-help guide, however, there is still much work to be done! First and foremost is to apply what you have learned in this book to real life. All of the treatments, therapies, and techniques are useless after all if you don't actively continue to practice them. When in doubt, feel free to return to this self-help guide and use it as a reference.

Maintain What You Have Learned

In any journey, there are bound to be several ups and downs. Chances are you will experience at least one relapse. There will be days when you desperately want to give up. There will be times when tackling your OCD seems an insurmountable task. It is during these critical times that we urge you not to give up! Instead of writing these experiences off as failures, use them as learning experiences. For example, if you do relapse, consider why this happened. Additionally, what could you do to prevent another relapse in the future?

Remember that you do not have to walk this path alone. If you feel overwhelmed, reach out to a Psychiatrist, Therapist, support group, or loved one. A complete list of resources can be found in chapter 16 of this book.

More likely than not, you will always have Obsessive-Compulsive Disorder. No amount of medication, therapies, or techniques will change that. However, this does not mean that your OCD should define you. Rather, by utilizing the therapies and techniques in this book (along with other sources at your disposal such as a Psychiatrist, Therapist, or the support of a loved one), it is our hope that you will take back control of your life and define yourself by your values and aspirations instead.

To this end, we wish you the best of luck on your journey and are so glad you let us take it with you!

Chapter 16: How to Get Help

Resources for Individuals with OCD

The path to overcoming your OCD can be a long and arduous one, filled with both triumphs and setbacks. The good news, however, is that you don't have to make this journey alone. Whether you are looking to find a therapist, support group, or additional information, we hope that you will find the following resources a helpful place to start.

Where Can I Find Additional Information?

Both the International OCD Foundation and the National Alliance on Mental Illness (NAMI) are well-recognized organizations that offer a wealth of resources to those with OCD and other mental illnesses.

The International OCD Foundation offers a number of articles on OCD written by experts in the field. They also offer webinars and other educational materials for those who are interested. Given the number of resources they offer, this organization is an excellent place to start if you don't know where to turn. Visit their website to start exploring the resources they offer: International OCD Foundation | Home (iocdf.org).

The National Alliance on Mental Illness is an excellent resource if you are looking to find out more about other mental health conditions in addition to OCD. The organization provides mental health education, access to a video resource library, and online discussion groups. Additional information can be found on their website: Home | NAMI: National Alliance on Mental Illness.

Finding a Therapist, Psychiatrist, or Support Group

The International OCD Foundation offers a resource directory that can be used to find therapists, treatment programs, clinics, and support groups that specialize in Obsessive-Compulsive Disorder in your area. More information can be found on their website:

International OCD Foundation | Home (iocdf.org)

Home - Hoarding (iocdf.org)

The NAMI has support groups across the U.S. that meet weekly, biweekly, or monthly depending on the location. They also offer a Family Support Group for family members, significant others, and friends of people with mental health conditions. If you are interested, take a moment to find a support group near you: Support Groups | NAMI: National Alliance on Mental Illness.

NAMI also has a HelpLine that can be reached Monday through Friday, from 10 am-6 pm, ET. The HelpLine is unique in that it is a peer-support service. It can be reached by phone or email and provides information, support, and resource referrals to those with mental health conditions, their family, friends, and caregivers.

Phone: 1-800-950-NAMI (6264)

Email: info@nami.org

It's important to note that the NAMI HelpLine is not a crisis line or suicide prevention line. It is also unable to provide mental health counseling or referrals to mental health providers. If you feel that you are in crisis, please see our list of resources below. If you need help immediately, call 911 or the National Suicide Prevention Lifeline at 800-273-TALK (8255).

Reaching Out in Times of Crisis

If you feel that you are in crisis, don't be afraid to reach out for help! NAMI offers a guide titled "Navigating a

Mental Health Crisis" on their website. The 33 page PDF is a helpful resource for those experiencing a mental health crisis: Navigating a Mental Health Crisis | NAMI: National Alliance on Mental Illness.

If you are in crisis and need to speak with someone immediately, the National Suicide Prevention Lifeline is staffed by trained crisis counselors and is available 24/7. To speak with a crisis counselor, call 800-273-TALK (8255).

If you are not comfortable speaking with someone over the phone, you can also communicate with a trained crisis counselor via text message. The Crisis Text Line is available 24/7 and can be accessed by texting NAMI to 741-741.

Both the National Suicide Prevention Lifeline and the Crisis Text Line are completely confidential and free.

Chapter 17: Resources for Family Members

How to Support Your Loved One

If you are the family member or loved one of a person who has been diagnosed with OCD, you have likely asked yourself, "How can I support them?" or "What can I do to help?"

Fortunately, there are a wealth of resources available to help guide you through this process. Before you can support your loved one, however, you need to have an understanding of what Obsessive-Compulsive Disorder is. By reading this book, you have taken that first, critical step in helping your loved one. However, we encourage you to continue learning everything you can about OCD. The more you know, the more you will be able to help your loved one. To this end, we have provided a list of resources below.

If you are the parent of a child with OCD and are interested in finding additional information or resources, we have included a section dedicated to this topic as well. Here, you will also find resources for PANDAS/PANS.

When supporting your loved one, it may also be helpful to talk with other families going through the same thing. Support groups can be helpful in this regard and may even provide opportunities to get help and support for yourself as well.

Helpful Resources

Where Can I Find More Information About OCD?

If you're unsure of where to start, the International OCD Foundation is an excellent resource. In addition to providing an overview of what OCD is and how it is treated, the organization has a page dedicated to helping the family members of people with OCD. The site provides access to online articles written by experts in the field and an online library.

Topics covered on the site include learning how to recognize and reduce "family accommodation behaviors", and how to help a family member who refuses to seek treatment for their condition.

International OCD Foundation for Families: International OCD Foundation | Families and OCD (iocdf.org).

International OCD Foundation Book/Media Library: International OCD Foundation | Books and Multimedia About OCD and Related Disorders (iocdf.org)

,

My Child Was Diagnosed with OCD – How Can I Support Them?

Being the parent of a child with OCD can be especially challenging. Fortunately, the International OCD Foundation offers a host of resources dedicated to helping children who have been diagnosed with OCD and their parents.

In particular, the organization provides educational material for children and provides advice on what to do if their OCD begins impacting their experience at school. There are also educational OCD cartoons, comics, and videos that can be used to enhance your child's learning experience.

If you are unsure of how you should approach the topic of OCD with your child or teen, the International OCD Foundation can be a helpful guide. Other topics include how to communicate effectively with your child's therapist, doctor, and school. The book and multimedia library also contains a variety of resources for children and their families.

International OCD Foundation for Kids and Families: Home - OCD in Kids (iocdf.org)

International OCD Foundation Book/Media Library: International OCD Foundation | Books and Multimedia About OCD and Related Disorders (iocdf.org)

OCD Cartoons: OCD Cartoons - OCD in Kids (iocdf.org)

The International OCD Foundation's Resource Directory can also be used to locate a therapist for your child. Additional information can be found here: How Do I Find the Right Therapist for My Child? - OCD in Kids (iocdf.org).

Resources for PANDAS/PANS

The onset of Pediatric Autoimmune Neuropsychiatric Disorders Associated with Streptococcal Infections (PANDAS) or Pediatric Acute-onset Neuropsychiatric Syndrome (PANS) is often sudden and debilitating. If you believe your child may have PANDAS or PANS, prompt medical attention is necessary. Therefore, we highly recommend reaching out to your child's pediatrician as soon as possible.

To learn more about PANDAS and PANS, we recommend taking a look at the resources provided by the International OCD Foundation and the PANDAS Network.

International OCD Foundation PANDAS/PANS: Signs & Symptoms of PANDAS/PANS - OCD in Kids (iocdf.org)

PANDAS Network: What is PANDAS/PANS/AE? | PANDAS Network

PANDAS Network Treatment Options: Treatment | PANDAS Network

Locating a Support Group

Support groups provide an invaluable opportunity to share your experience in a safe, non-judgmental environment with other families going through similar situations. Additionally, it gives you the chance to obtain insights and advice from your peers.

While it is important to care for your loved one, it is also important to take care of yourself as well. Certain support groups, such as those run by NAMI, can help empower you through experience sharing and promote healthy coping skills. NAMI's Family Support Groups are free, confidential, and are led by family members of individuals with mental health conditions. Sessions are held weekly, biweekly, or monthly depending on location and typically last 60-90 minutes. To locate a support group near you, visit NAMI's website: NAMI Family Support Group | NAMI: National Alliance on Mental Illness.

The International OCD Foundation also offers support groups for those with OCD and their loved ones. Support groups may be location-specific or held remotely via phone or online. Additional information can be found on their website: International OCD Foundation | Support Groups (iocdf.org).

Conclusion

Congratulations on making it through to the end of *The OCD Workbook*. While OCD is a chronic, life-long condition, we hope that you can use the tools and strategies provided in this self-help guide to break the cycle of your obsessions and compulsions and take back control of your life.

However, this is far from the last step of your journey. Going forward, you must continue to apply what you have learned in this book to real life. All of the treatments, therapies, and techniques are useless after all if you don't actively continue to practice them. If you need a refresher or are unsure of where to turn, don't be afraid to return to this self-help guide. We also encourage you to explore the resources provided in chapters 16 and 17 as well.

With that being said, we want to thank you for taking the time to work your way through this self-help guide. We hope that you found it helpful and informative and wish you the best of luck in your future endeavors.

Finally, if you found this book useful in any way, a review on Amazon is always appreciated!

References

Abramowitz, Jonathan. "Hypochondriasis: What Is It
and How Do You Treat It?" *Beyond OCD*, 30 Mar.
2018, beyondocd.org/expert-
perspectives/articles/hypochondriasis-what-is-it-
and-how-do-you-treat-it.

Ackerman, Courtney. "25 CBT Techniques and
Worksheets for Cognitive Behavioral Therapy."
PositivePsychology.com, 16 Oct. 2020,
positivepsychology.com/cbt-cognitive-behavioral-
therapy-techniques-worksheets/.

"ACT vs. CBT: What's the Difference?" *The Chelsea
Psychology Clinic*, 16 Aug. 2019,
www.thechelseapsychologyclinic.com/therapy/act
-vs-cbt/.

"Anxiety Disorders." *NAMI*, Dec. 2017,
www.nami.org/About-Mental-Illness/Mental-
Health-Conditions/Anxiety-Disorders.

Carey, Patrick. "What Is Exposure and Response
Prevention (ERP) Therapy? Why ERP For OCD
Treatment?" *NOCD*, 3 Nov. 2020,

www.treatmyocd.com/blog/what-exactly-is-
   exposure-and-response-prevention-erp.

Cherry, Kendra. "How Cognitive Behavior Therapy
   Works." *Verywell Mind*, 13 June 2020,
   www.verywellmind.com/what-is-cognitive-
   behavior-therapy-2795747.

Cherry, Kendra. "The Fight-or-Flight Response
   Prepares Your Body to Take Action." *Verywell
   Mind*, 18 Aug. 2019,
   www.verywellmind.com/what-is-the-fight-or-
   flight-response-2795194.

Chowdhury, Madhuleena. "ACT Therapy: The Theory
   Behind Acceptance and Commitment Therapy."
   PositivePsychology.com, 1 Sept. 2020,
   positivepsychology.com/act-therapy/.

"Cognitive Behavioral Therapy Exercises." *Cognitive
   Behavioral Therapy Los Angeles*, 2020,
   cogbtherapy.com/cognitive-behavioral-therapy-
   exercises.

"Cognitive Defusion." *The University of Sydney*,
   www.sydney.edu.au/content/dam/students/docu

ments/counselling-and-mental-health-
support/cognitive-defusion.pdf.

"Cognitive Restructuring (Guide)." *Therapist Aid*,
Therapist Aid, 26 Feb. 2017,
www.therapistaid.com/therapy-guide/cognitive-
restructuring.

Cuncic, Arlin. "The Best Types of Therapy to Treat
Anxiety." *Verywell Mind*, 30 June 2020,
www.verywellmind.com/anxiety-therapy-
4692759.

D'Arcy-Sharpe, Ann-Marie. "A Guide to OCD Triggers."
Impulse, 14 Dec. 2020, impulsetherapy.com/a-
guide-to-ocd-triggers/.

D'Arcy-Sharpe, Ann-Marie. "Your Guide to Mindfulness
for OCD." *Impulse*, 26 Nov. 2020,
impulsetherapy.com/your-guide-to-mindfulness-
for-ocd/.

"Depression." *NAMI*, Aug. 2017, www.nami.org/About-
Mental-Illness/Mental-Health-
Conditions/Depression.

"Differential Diagnosis of OCD or PANDAS/PANS."
     OCD in Kids, 9 July 2015,
     kids.iocdf.org/professionals/md/ocd-or-pandas/.

"Educational Resources." *International OCD
     Foundation*, 18 Sept. 2020, iocdf.org/ocd-finding-
     help/other-resources/.

Eisler, Melissa. "Ease Anxiety with These 5 Visualization
     Techniques." *Mindful Minutes*, 6 June 2018,
     mindfulminutes.com/ease-anxiety-with-
     visualization-techniques/.

Empower Your Mind Therapy. "Anxiety Relief Using
     DBT Skills and Mindfulness: DBT Therapy NYC."
     Empower Your Mind Therapy, Empower Your
     Mind Therapy, 18 Dec. 2019,
     eymtherapy.com/blog/anxiety-relief-dbt-skills/.

Hershfield, Jon, and Tom Corboy. "Mindfulness and
     Cognitive Behavioral Therapy for OCD."
     International OCD Foundation, 5 Aug. 2020,
     iocdf.org/expert-opinions/mindfulness-and-
     cognitive-behavioral-therapy-for-ocd/.

"Hypochondriasis." *OCD Resource Center*, 20 Dec.
     2014, www.ocdhope.com/hypochondriasis/.

Janette. "DBT Mindfulness Exercises." *Mindfulness4U*, 26 Jan. 2019, mindfulness4u.org/dbt-mindfulness-exercises/.

Kelly, Owen. "Do They Know What Causes Obsessive-Compulsive Disorder?" *Verywell Mind*, 26 July 2020, www.verywellmind.com/causes-of-ocd-2510476.

Kelly, Owen. "How to Improve Your OCD Self-Help Strategy With Relaxation Techniques." *Verywell Mind*, 15 Dec. 2020, www.verywellmind.com/relaxation-is-an-essential-ocd-self-help-technique-2510635.

Kelly, Owen. "Stress When You Have OCD Can Make Your Symptoms Worse." *Verywell Mind*, 15 Dec. 2020, www.verywellmind.com/understanding-ocd-and-stress-2510559.

Langham, R.Y. "Hyper-Responsibility & OCD: What Does It All Mean?" *Impulse*, 10 Dec. 2020, impulsetherapy.com/hyper-responsibility-ocd-what-does-it-all-mean/.

Moore, Catherine. "21 ACT Worksheets and Ways to Apply Acceptance & Commitment Therapy."

PositivePsychology.com, 9 Nov. 2020,
positivepsychology.com/act-worksheets/.

Munford, Paul. "Self-Directed Treatment for OCD: The
Irony of Doing the Opposite." *International OCD
Foundation*, 14 Aug. 2020, iocdf.org/expert-
opinions/expert-opinion-self-directed-erp/.

"NAMI HelpLine." *NAMI*, 2020, www.nami.org/help.

Neziroglu, Fugen. "Hoarding: The Basics." *Anxiety and
Depression Association of America, ADAA*,
adaa.org/understanding-anxiety/obsessive-
compulsive-disorder-ocd/hoarding-basics.

"OCD Symptoms: OCD-Related Hoarding." *Beyond
OCD*, 2 Apr. 2018, beyondocd.org/information-
for-individuals/symptoms/ocd-related-hoarding.

"PANS/PANDAS." *PPN*, 25 June 2020,
www.pandasppn.org/what-are-pans-pandas/.

Penzel, Fred. "Call Me Irresponsible: OCD and Hyper-
Responsibility." *Western Suffolk Psychological
Services*, Western Suffolk Psychological Services,
14 Feb. 2020, www.wsps.info/articles/call-me-
irresponsible-ocd-and-hyper-responsibility.

Phillipson. "Comorbidity and OCD." *Made of Millions Foundation*, www.madeofmillions.com/ocd/comorbidity-and-ocd.

"Related Conditions: Disorders That May Co-Exist with OCD." *Beyond OCD*, 1 Apr. 2018, beyondocd.org/ocd-facts/related-conditions.

Riemann, Bradley. "Cognitive-Behavioral Treatment for Obsessive-Compulsive Disorder." *Psychiatric Times*, 1 Aug. 2006, www.psychiatrictimes.com/view/cognitive-behavioral-treatment-obsessive-compulsive-disorder.

Riemann, Bradley. "What Is Habituation And What Role Does It Play In OCD Treatment?" *Beyond OCD*, 30 Mar. 2018, beyondocd.org/expert-perspectives/articles/what-does-habituation-mean.

Schiffer, Molly. "Shedding Light on Health Anxiety OCD." *Sheppard Pratt*, 11 Aug. 2018, www.sheppardpratt.org/news-views/story/shedding light-on-health-anxiety-ocd/.

"Signs & Symptoms of PANDAS/PANS." *OCD in Kids*, 9 July 2015, kids.iocdf.org/professionals/md/pandas/.

Singer, Janet. "OCD and Hyper-Responsibility." *Mental Help OCD and HyperResponsibility Comments*, www.mentalhelp.net/blogs/ocd-and-hyper-responsibility/.

Singer, Janet. "OCD and Mindfulness." *Psych Central*, Psych Central, 17 May 2016, psychcentral.com/lib/ocd-and-mindfulness.

"Treating OCD With Cognitive Behavior Therapy (College Students)." *Beyond OCD*, 2 Apr. 2018, beyondocd.org/information-for-college-students/cognitive-behavior-therapy.

"Treatment of Hoarding Disorder." *Hoarding*, 6 Nov. 2017, hoarding.iocdf.org/professionals/treatment-of-hoarding-disorder/.

"Treatment." *OCD in Kids*, 9 July 2015,
      kids.iocdf.org/professionals/md/treatment/.

"Treatments for OCD." *Anxiety and Depression
      Association of America, ADAA*,
      adaa.org/understanding-anxiety/obsessive-
      compulsive-disorder-ocd/treatments-for-ocd.

Twohig, Michael. "What Is ACT?" *International OCD
      Foundation*, 5 Aug. 2020, iocdf.org/expert-
      opinions/expert-opinion-what-is-act/.

Vidrine, Ryan. "Cognitive Defusion Techniques For
      OCD And BDD." *NOCD*, 16 Dec. 2020,
      www.treatmyocd.com/blog/cognitive-defusion-
      and-ocd-techniques-that-are-easy-to-try.

Wignall, Nick. "Cognitive Restructuring: The Complete
      Guide to Changing Negative Thinking [2020]."
      Nick Wignall, 22 Oct. 2020,
      nickwignall.com/cognitive-restructuring/.

Manufactured by Amazon.ca
Bolton, ON